Health Care Today: Expanded Edition

Active Ingredients vs Placebo Ingredients

ReEnvision Press

Contents

Introduction	1
Chapter 0: The Ground Floor	6
Chapter 1	11
Chapter 2	16
Chapter 3	25
Chapter 4	31
Chapter 5	40
Chapter 6	48
Chapter 7	56
Chapter 8	65
Chapter 9	71
Chapter 10	81

Chapter 11: Example of a Healing Archetype? A Movie on YouTube 86

Finale: Not Everything is Rocket Science 88

Dedication 93

Video and Print Resources 96

Introduction

This Expanded Edition contains many images not found in the Kindle version.

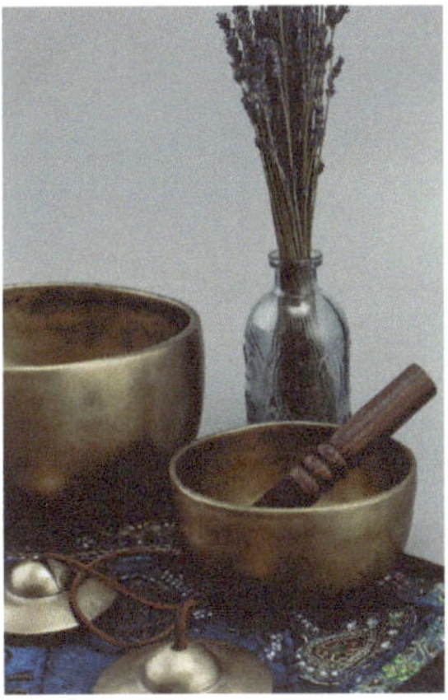

This author has worked as a paid and unpaid home health aid for many years.

He also started his own home health care company, at one point.

He was once a pre-med major at West Point, before switching to electrical engineering as a major. He was getting a grade of D in his boxing and gymnastics classes, and this was an impediment to having a stellar GPA that was required for medical school after completion of pre-med studies. His physical stature was such, in fact, that he was one of the very few cadets assigned to eat all of his dinner meals, for several months, with the members of the West Point football team, so that he would be provided with double "rations" of food. He also was assigned the sport of weight-lifting, his first year: all the other weight-lifters during the sport period, were, again, members of the football team. Finally, his first roommate, ever, was also a football team member.

He remembers having to attend "additional instruction", after academic classroom hours, in boxing. Had it not been for having had a U.S . Army Ranger School graduate, that first year, originally from New York City, as a squad leader –

a most rare scenario - he might well have not made it through the grueling four-year program.

***

He is no stranger to the medical ideas of our country, what with having visited his mother in three different "homes" and numerous hospitals, through the years, over five hundred times, total.

She is still alive, today, at the age of 86, a war refugee from the eastern-most part of Poland, coming to America at the age of twelve, via a two-week long steamship voyage, to Ellis Island.

***

This book is also dedicated to his Aunt Joly in Germany, whom he used to visit, when he lived in Bavaria for several years. She was a German medical doctor, also living in Bavaria.

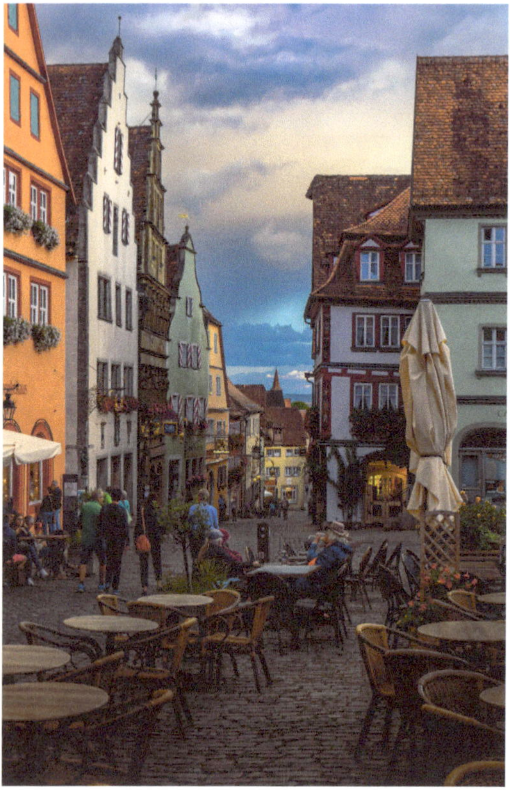

A town in Bavaria, Germany, not far from where this author and his aunt, a German medical doctor, lived.

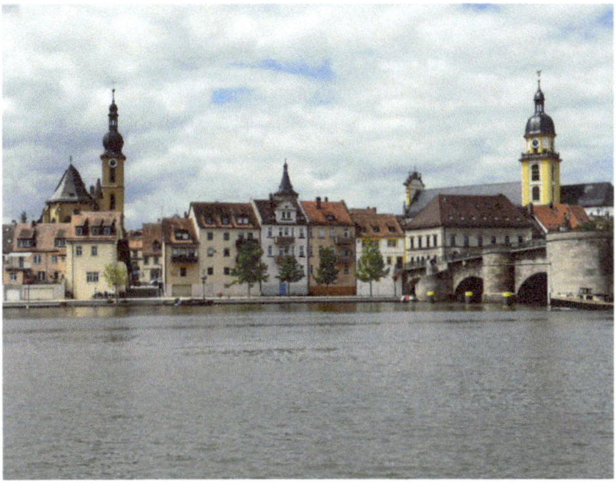

This is the Bavarian village where this author lived, for three years, when he was in his twenties. He dated a German citizen, who lived next door, for a year. He grew up hearing German spoken daily during his summers on his grandparent's farm, and attended a church each Sunday as a youth, where services were in German. His mother also spoke German.

Chapter O: The Ground Floor

Is our suffering all physical in nature?

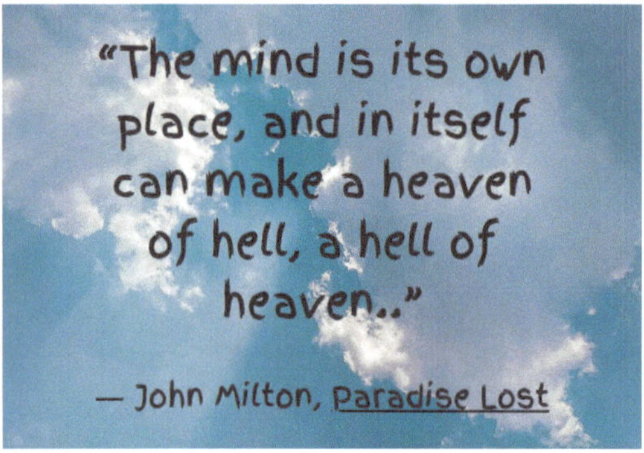

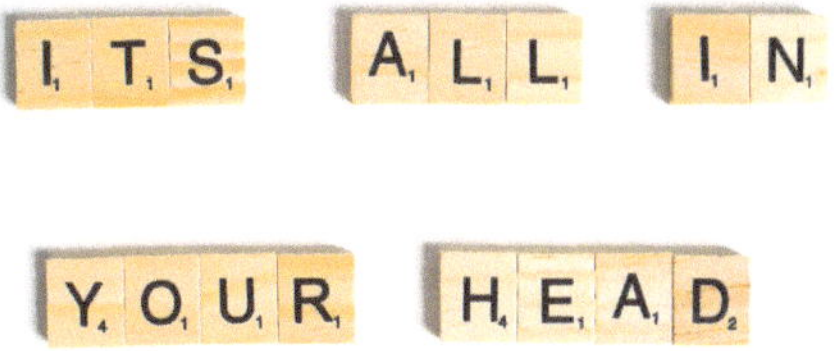

"Don't play head games with me?"

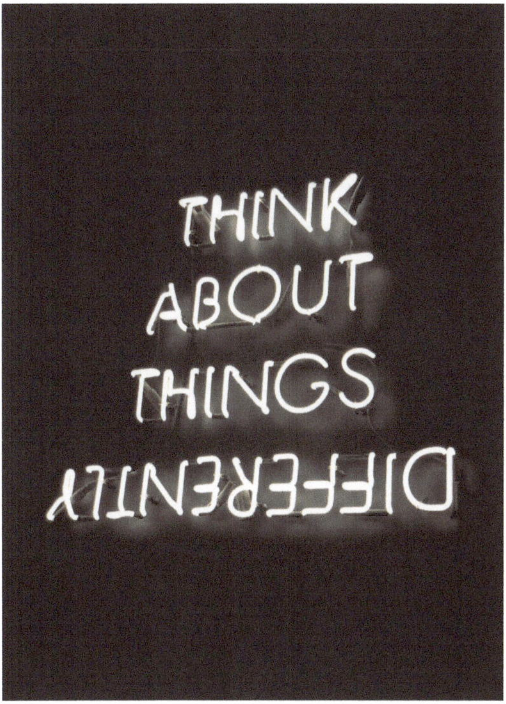

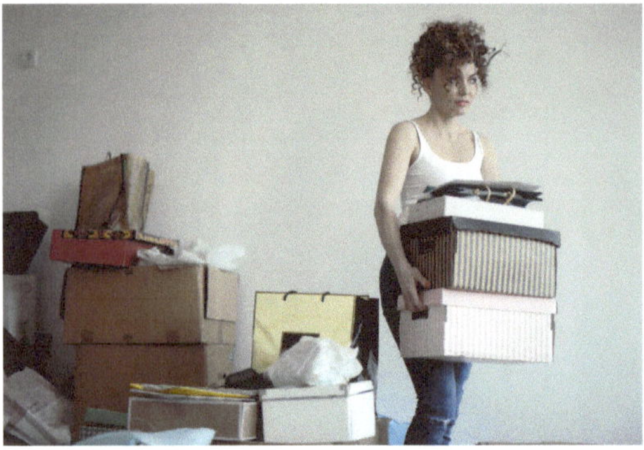

Are we moving, or is life moving us?

Might we consider Jack LaLanne?
"Jack LaLanne at Age 95":

https://youtu.be/AkdYrAQJu6g

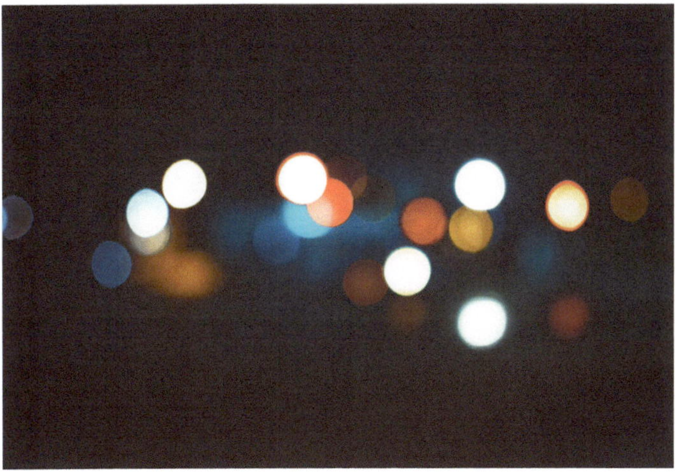

Chapter 1

We often hear the topic of stress bandied about, but we never examine what it is that makes us feel stressed!

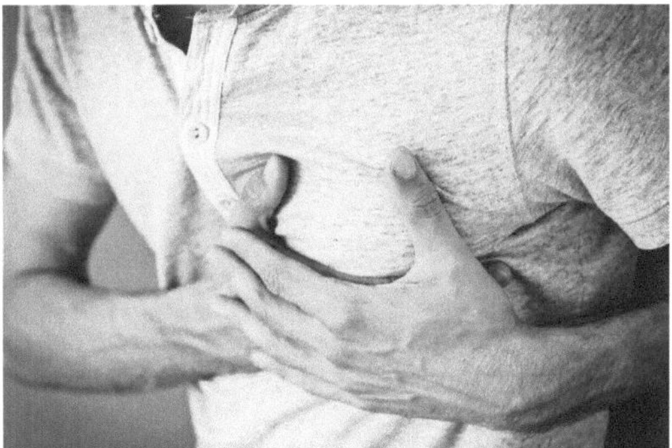

We have, though, heard the phrase, "stress kills".

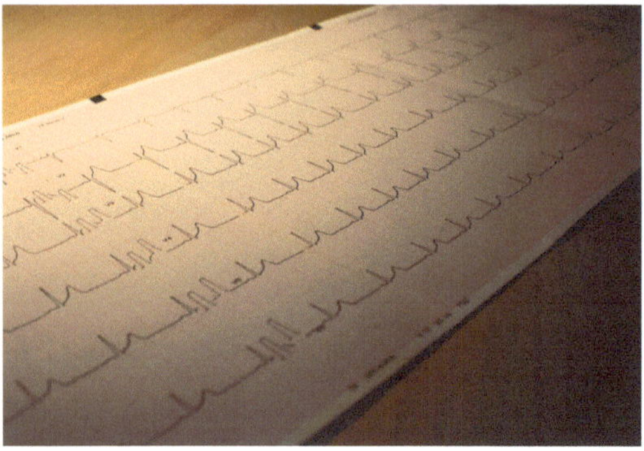

We've also heard the phrase, "What doesn't kill, you makes you stronger - but bears will kill you".

What if that bear is stress, and the attack of the bear, so to speak, is cumulative and slow in action, as if a slow form of cancer?

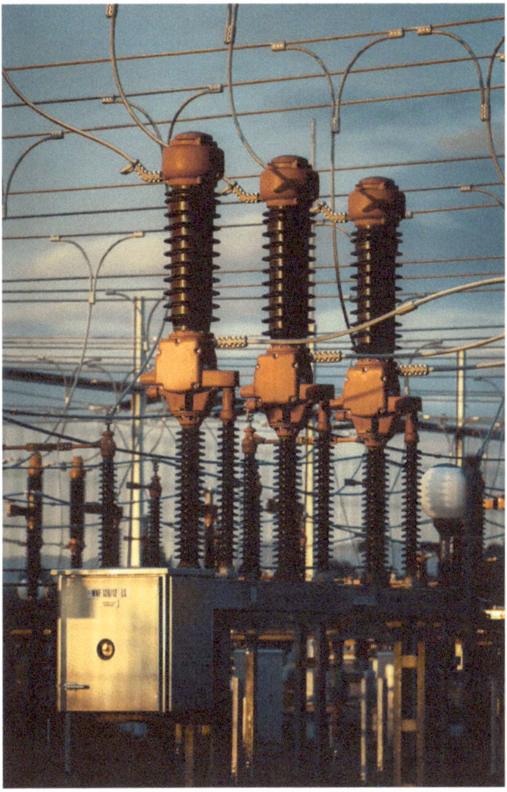

On the other hand, a magazine, "Forks Over Knives", has talked of how a many people have cholesterol-filled arteries, and yet, that this is not necessarily a big problem until one has a very difficult day – and then, all of a sudden – one has a sudden blockage or such, followed by a heart attack....

Another person has related his idea that heart attacks typically occur on a Monday. Why would that be, unless one may be very unhappy, going back to work on Mondays, and one's stress level, that day, is higher than on the other days? Perhaps one also had had an action-packed, stressful week-end, and also did not garner that much sleep.

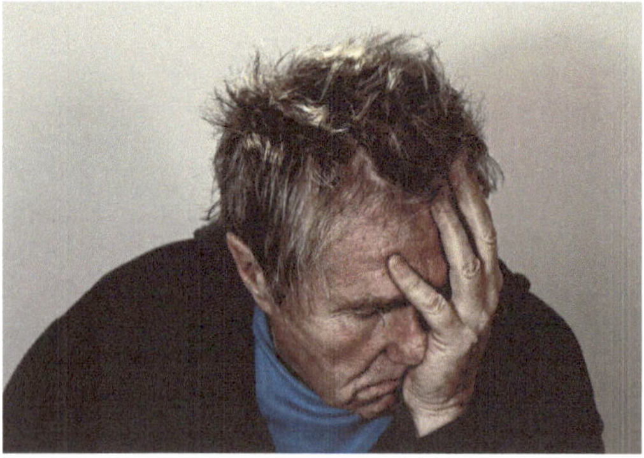

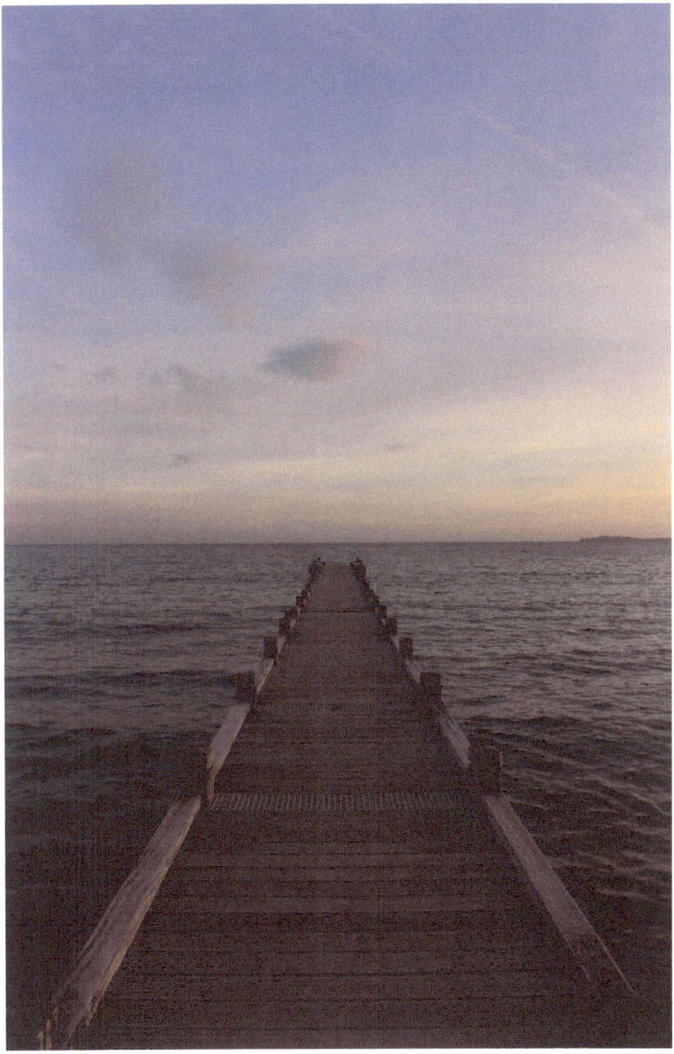

Chapter 2

Now, we might well ask, “Just what is stress”?

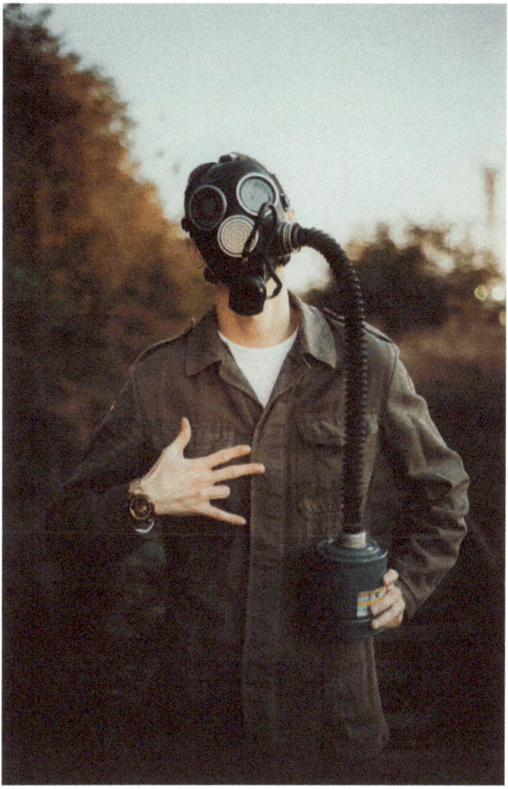

I think we need to delve into two key words:

Fear and anger.

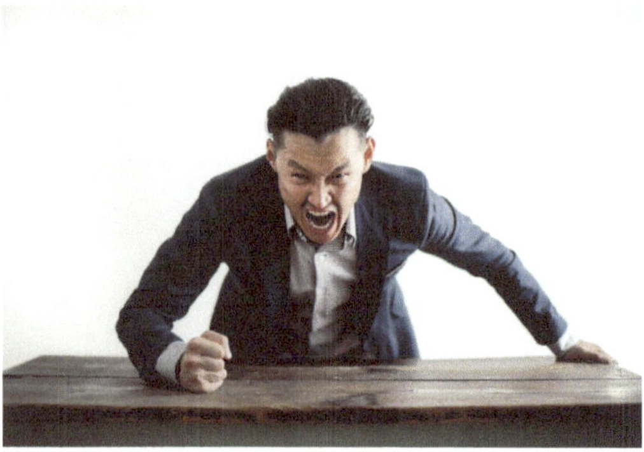

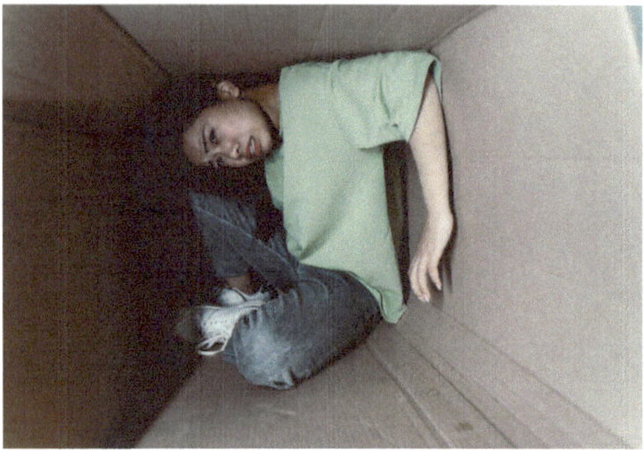

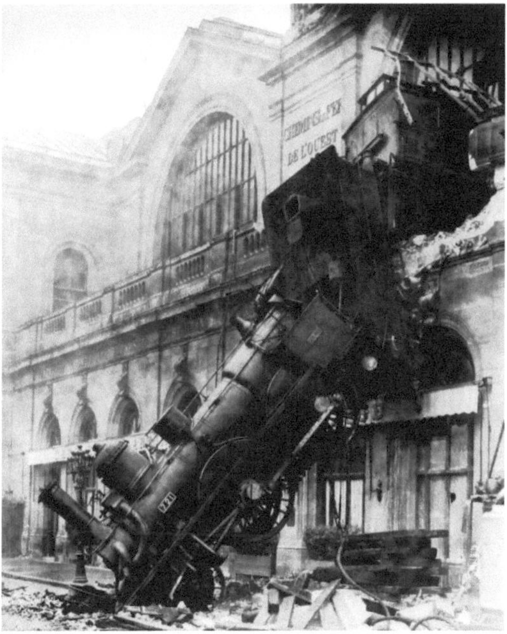

Might we consider: that if we have considerable fears – or engage in a considerable amount of catastrophizing, we might say – then surely we could call this “stress”.

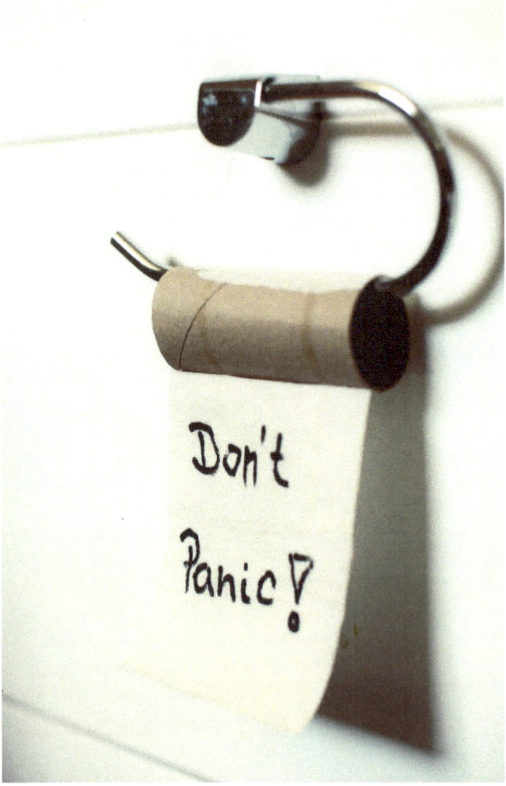

I won't try and discuss the impact on the chemicals in our body.

I don't think this is the most important focus, here.

Although we might consider the book, "The Relaxation Response", by Dr. Herbert Benson.

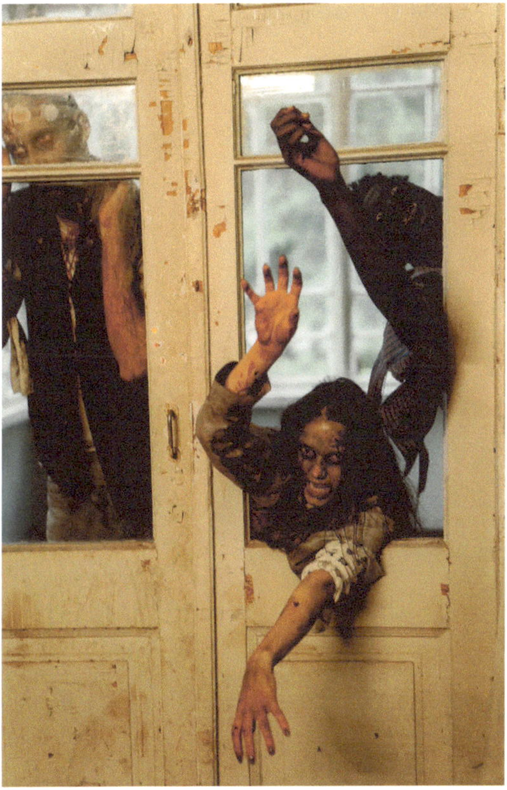

Not quite what the doctor ordered?

Might this "relaxing" be a way of reducing the impact of the anger and fear in our lives?

Might this thus be achieved through any number of ways, such as a relaxing bath, or a good walk, or even our favorite tranquilizer pill, or a comforting talk with someone? Or perhaps being apart from what was "triggering" the anger or fear in the first place? Hence, "unplugging", for a while, from the "triggers" which we say were "stressing" us?

Some have also turned to mindfulness meditation.

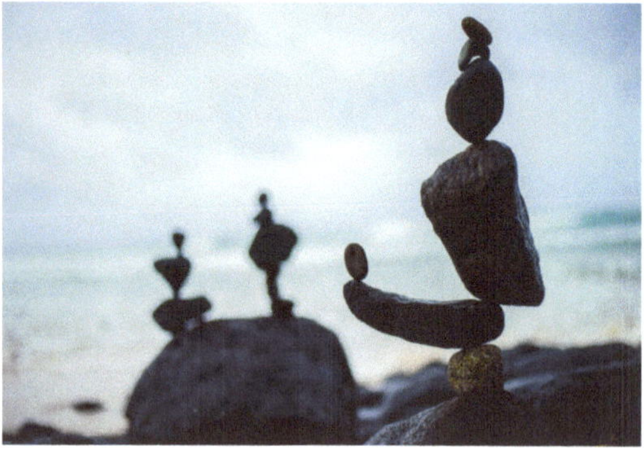

Might this be a way of "unplugging" from the triggering words we assign to the "trigger" events?

For, if we think less, we find the flow of "triggering" words acting upon us less, too?

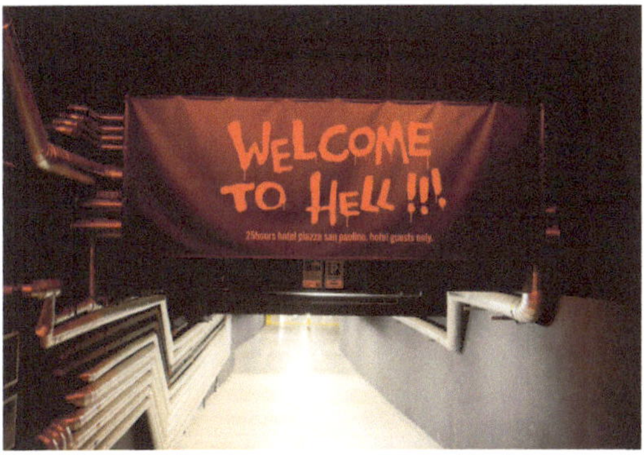

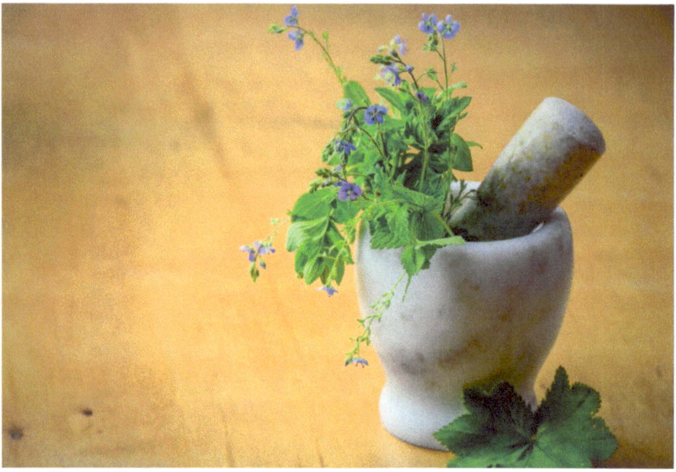

Chapter 3

There are those who say that heart disease, cancer, and stroke, are largely modern illnesses.

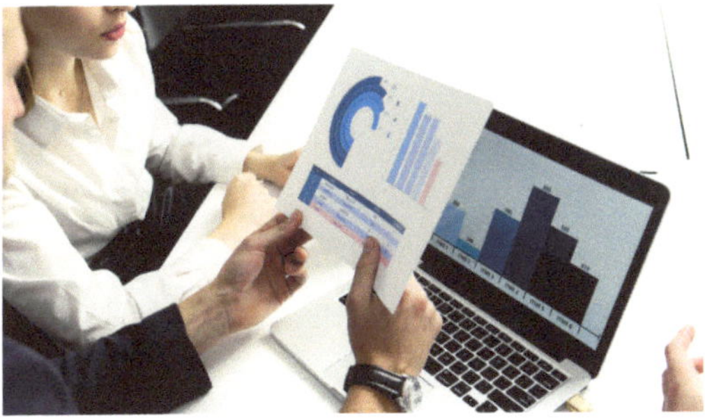

Let's not forget these items when we go on our picnic this weekend!

Might this be said, because the levels of stress – the levels of anger and fear that we have – may well be at unprecedented levels, too?

The presence of marked anger and fear surely wear upon our bodies, over time: and eventually, something must "give":

In the way of our hearts, our body cells, and in our blood vessels – including our brain's blood vessels.

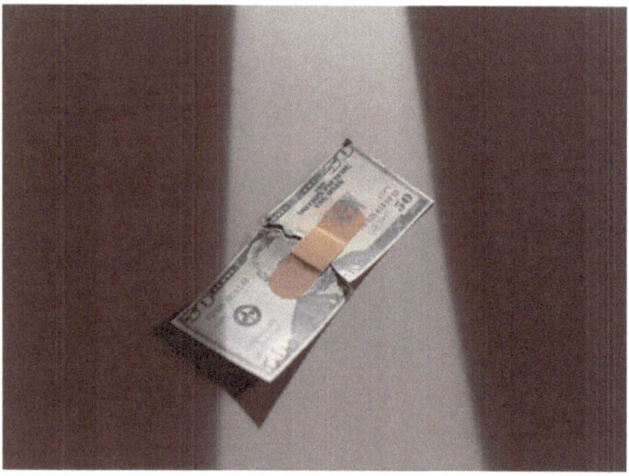

Pema Chodron, the Buddhist nun, has talked about the importance of working on our anger and fear.

Now, cognitive therapists also are attempting to modify how we feel, by modifying our thinking.

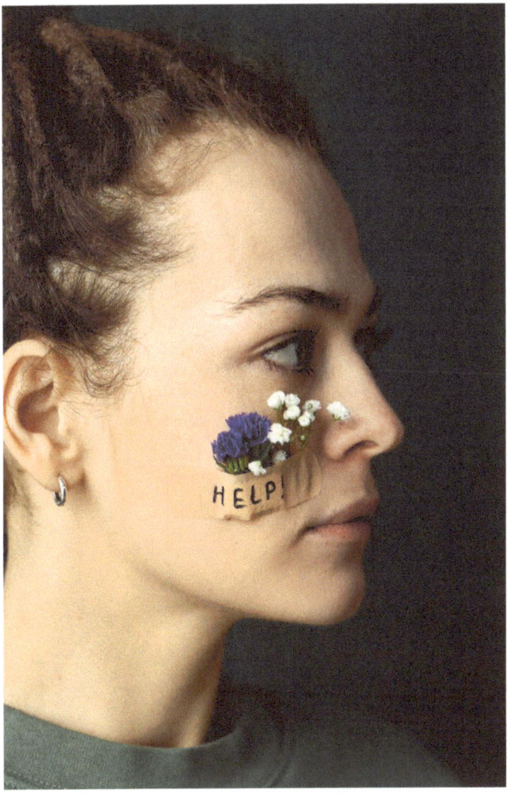

Perhaps the two words, anger and fear, are most succinct, if we are wondering just where the focus is best put, in modifying what produces these "feelings"?

We could consider the ideas from Rational Emotive Therapy, Reality Therapy, or Cognitive Therapy, for instance, noting that Dr. David D. Burns had attempted to help people modify their thinking so that they felt happier – we might say, felt less anger and fear, to put it in tight focus.

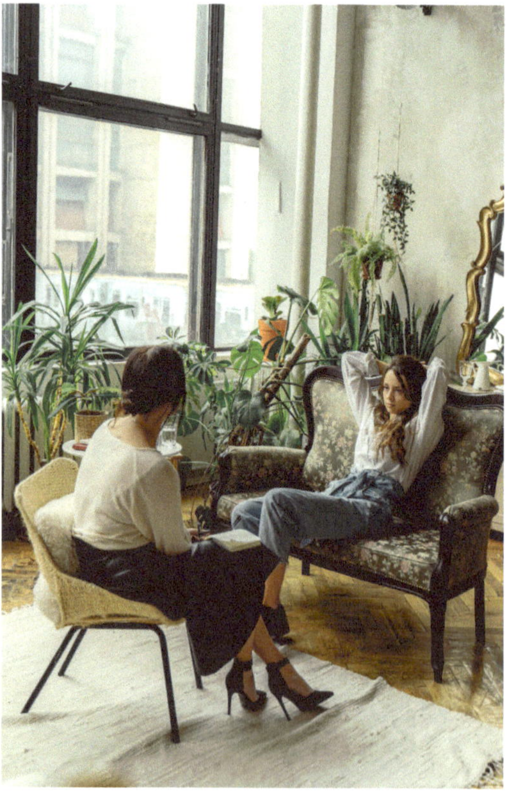

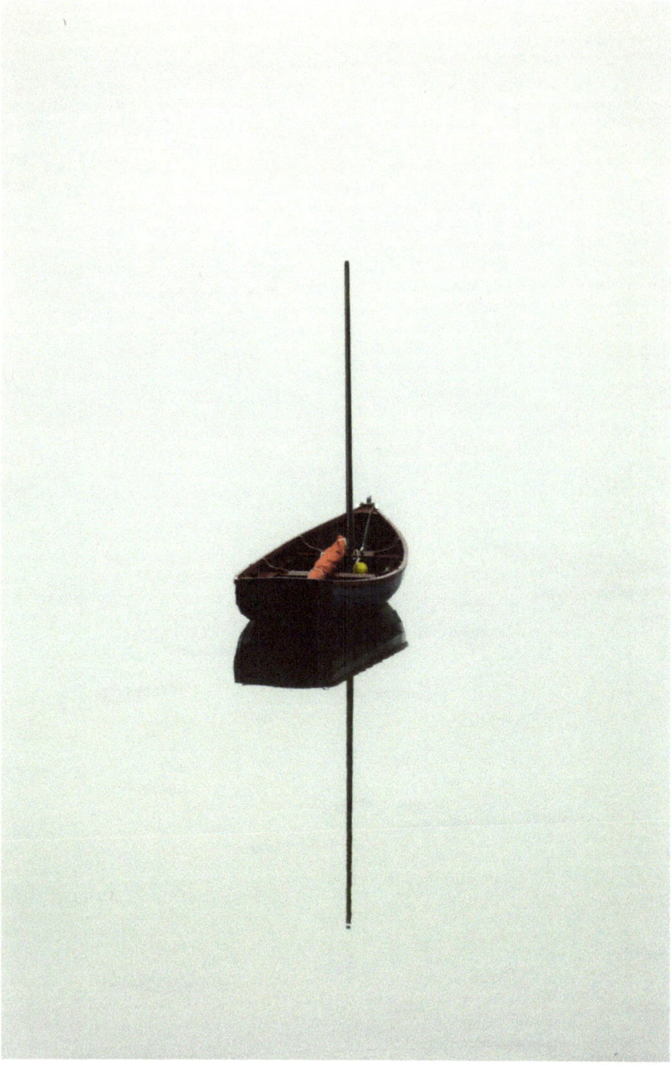

Chapter 4

One has to wonder: perhaps many – if even more than "many" – people have not found wholly satisfying results from what we may refer to as "modern medicine", other than if surgery is involved for a broken bone, say, or other clear-cut "mechanical" problem, is because the issues of anger and fear are not being sufficiently addressed.

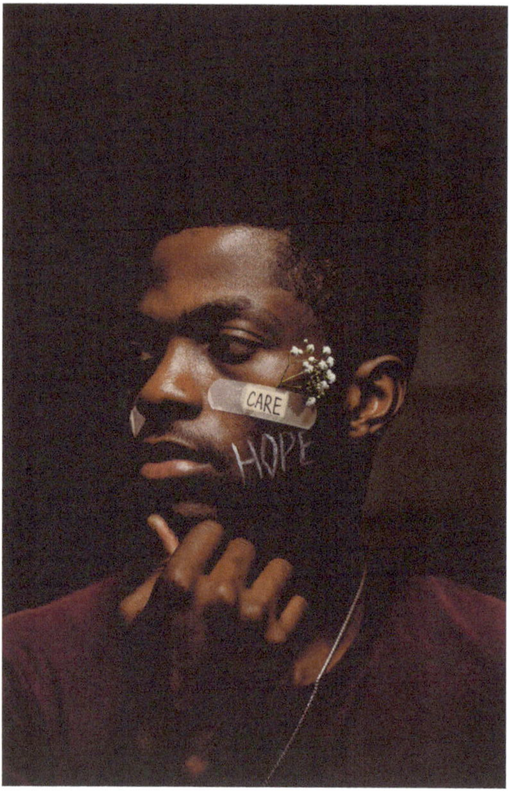

We often hear, for instance, the phrase, "psychosomatic" illness.

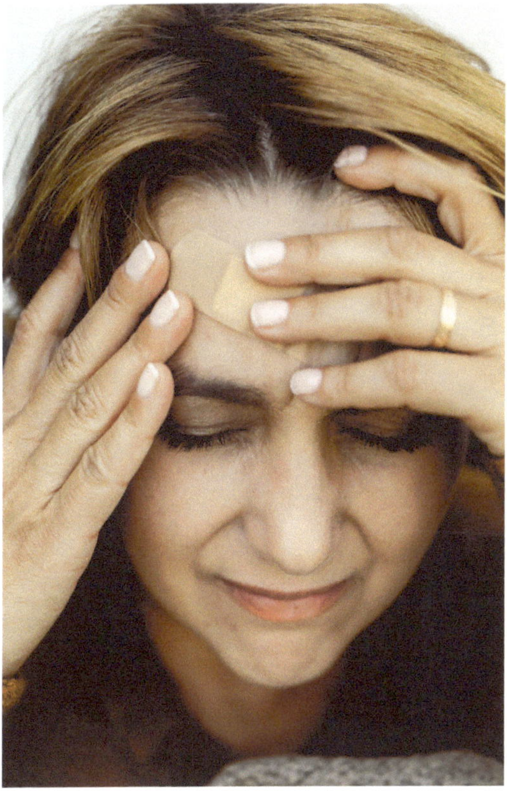

What if most all illnesses are almost entirely due to what this phrase, "psyche", is referring to? The component of what is going on, in our psyches – our brains – as per the thinking involved – and in turn, the anger and fears in ourselves?

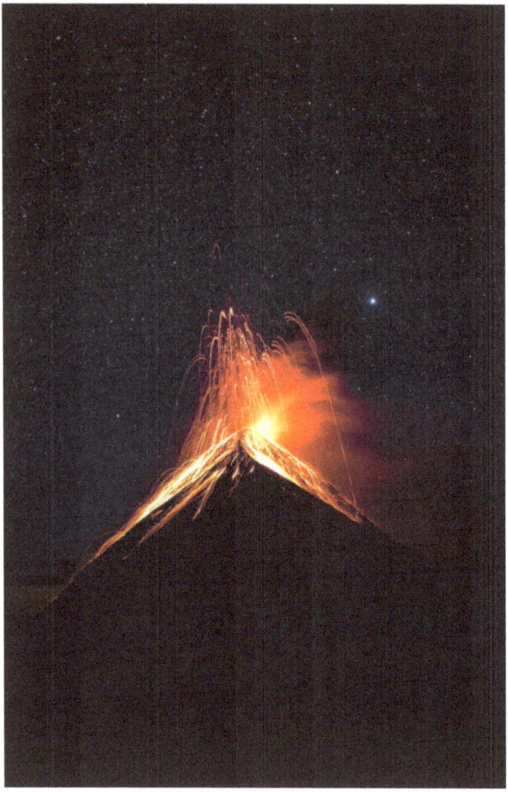

Indeed, do we remember the book, "Think and Grow Rich", by Napoleon Hill?

What if we were to modify the title to say, "Think and Grow More Physically Healthy"?

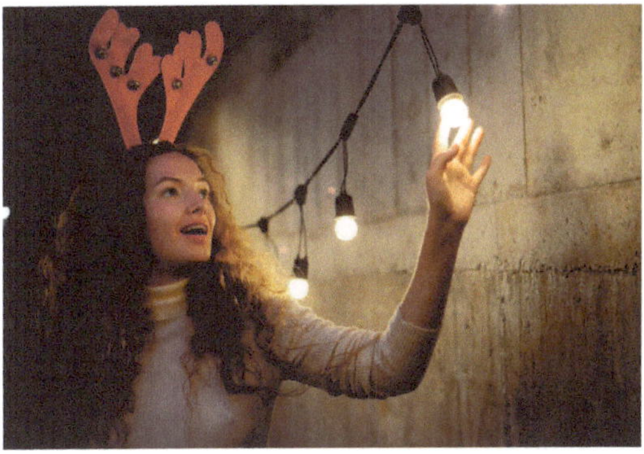

Let's see what's happening?

Or, "Think and Grow Less Angry and Fearful", as the antecedent to being healthier?

Consider, too:

We hear of "tainted" food; we experience "tainted" drugs, too, at times; we have "tainted" air to deal with; and neighborhoods which are "tainted" with crime and noise.

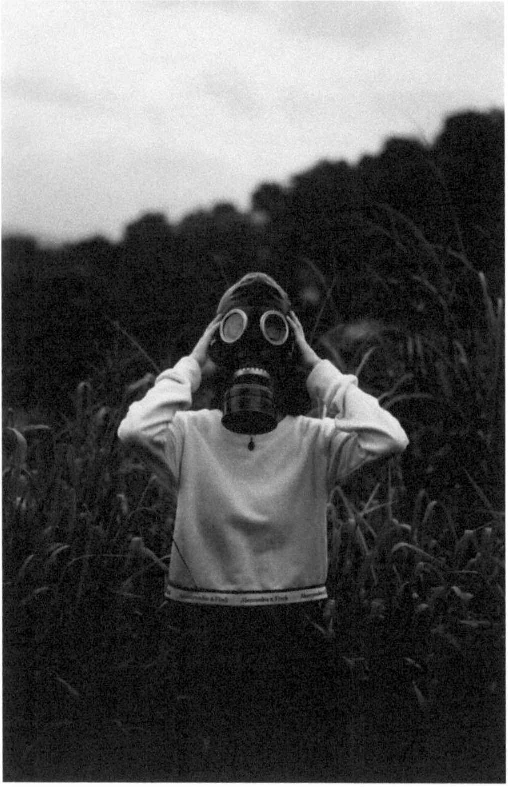

Indeed, in the early days of moonshine-making, car radiators were sometimes used in the process of making this moonshine, and the alcohol, then, was unfortunately "tainted" by lead in these radiators.

To put it in a nutshell, could our health often be "tainted" by "tainted" thinking, and our thinking, in turn, be "tainted" by "tainted" words, phrases, and premises?

If we "treat" the "tainted" thinking, we may well treat the "tainted" emotions, and in turn, improve our "tainted" health...

We have heard, too, "garbage in, garbage out".

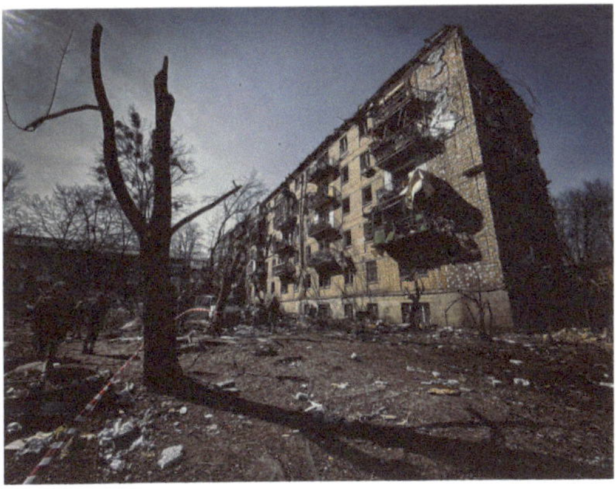

Might we say, too, "Garbage words in, Garbage Emotions Created, and Garbage Health, Out"?

This, of course, is assuming – a big assumption, these days – that our environments are not so toxically-laden with crime, noise, rushing, and too many novelties "per square foot" – that we are as overloaded as a young infant who is bewildered by noise, too much bright light, and not enough sleep...

Sort of like cooking something in a pressure cooker: the pressure cooker makes everything happen "more intensely", we might say. It acts like a catalyst to whatever is already there.

Just like the high decibel music, crowds, and more, in a rock concert arena.

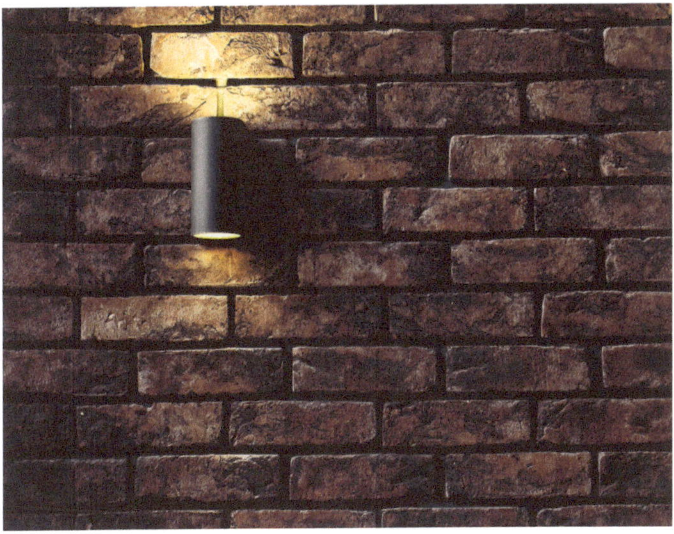

Chapter 5

We might now ask, what the definitions of tranquilizers and placebos are, finally.

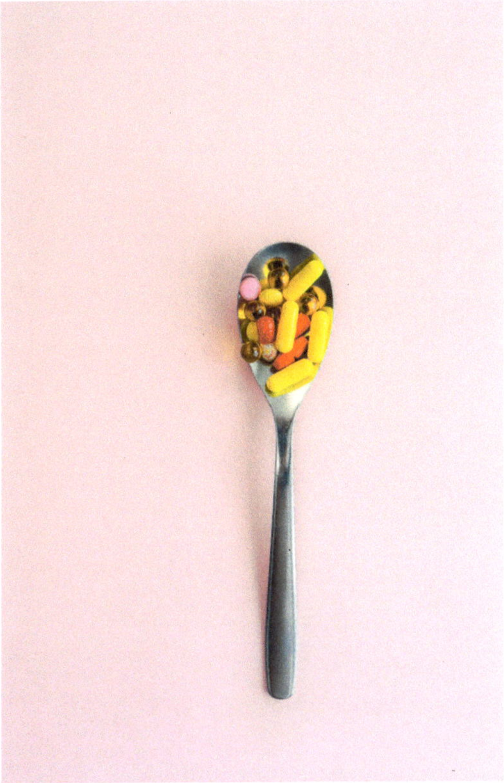

Time for our chill pill?

If we are not addressing the root causes of anything, everything else is surely not going to be having that much effect.

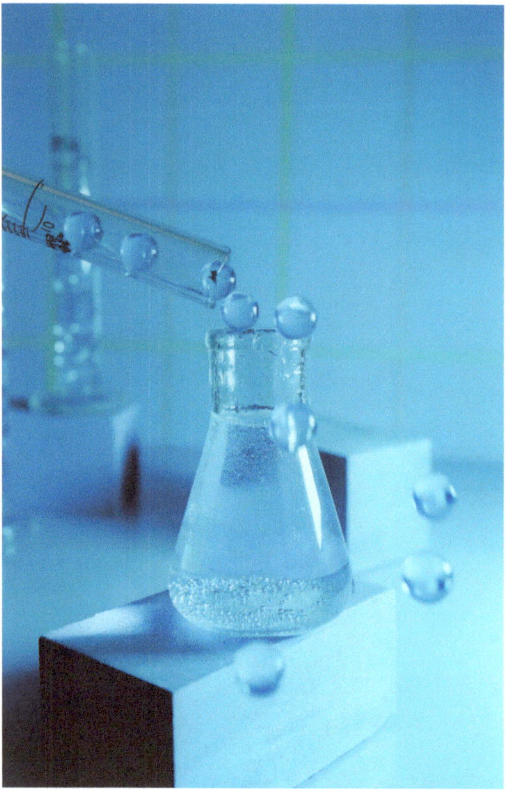

Is it rocket science that we are unhappier than ever? Maybe in ten thousand years, we will have the molecular structure of The Rat Race figured out?

We might thus even speculate, that whatever does not address the anger and fear which in turn generates stress, and then impacts our physical bodies, is a form of a placebo:

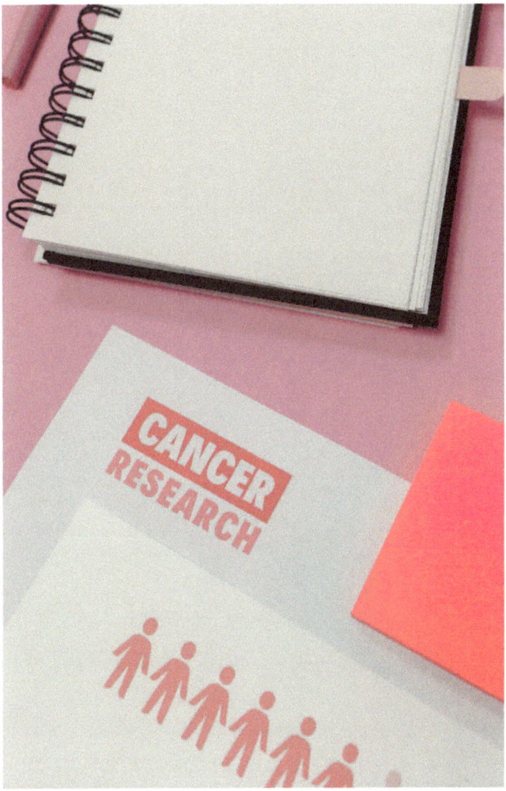

We will never cure cancer until we cure bill-cancer, boss-cancer, toxic-housing cancer, and fear-of-death-cancer?

Yes, placebos are medicine, we might conclude, inasmuch as hope is very beneficial; so too, is anything that is distracting.

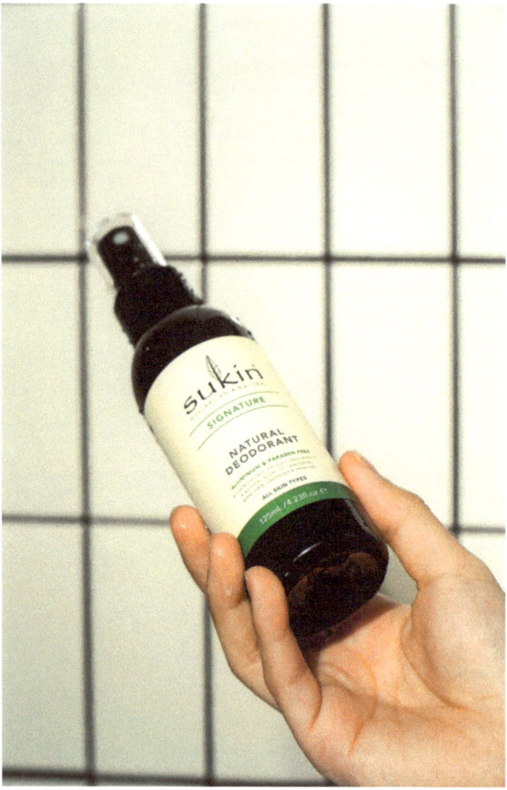

This substance will deodorize our anger and fear, but will it treat the roots or merely do a touchup?

Might the operative elements of a placebo, then, be hope and distraction?

These might be partial cures, but not a longer-lasting, and more thorough-going remedy.

Yes, hope has the effect of reducing our fears: We are hoping that something will happen to change one or more aspects of our lives, and the very act of anticipating a possible "cure" in future circumstances, reduces our worry – our fear, if you will, over those possible future experiences.

The trouble is, perhaps, that hope waxes and wanes. It could be described as "fickle". It does not remain, permanently, nor to the same extent, hour by hour, day by day.

If we want temporary solutions, we apply a band-aid solution – and alas, band-aids eventually lose their "stickiness", and fall off, and then, that is the end of the band-aid's treatment.

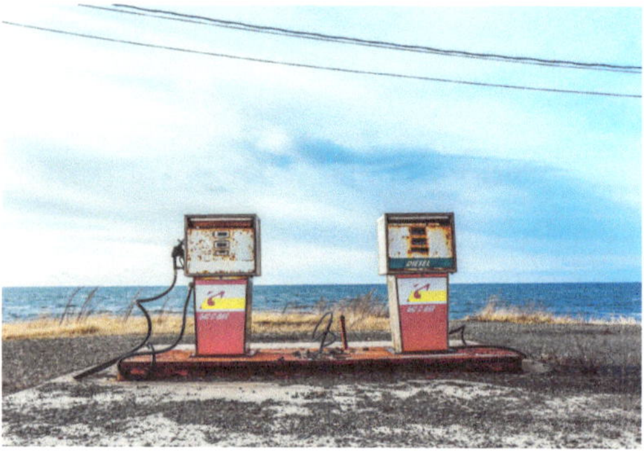

"Man does not live by gas alone".

The same, for a chemical tranquilizer; or for use of food; or sleep; or meditating; or a variety of distractive activities; or for "hope"; or meditation; or isolating; or sleeping, arguably a form of isolating – isolating from both environmental triggers and the words in our head, which are also triggers, one might say.

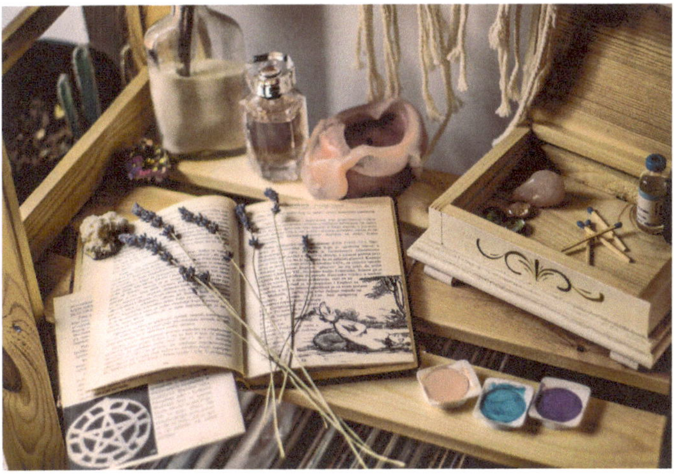

Chapter 6

Indeed, if we think of the proverbial Thanksgiving Dinner as prepared by Grandma, might the "medicine" in a wonderful Thanksgiving Dinner, be the application of "Grandma-Medicine": the elements of "Comfort(ing) Food", the example of Comforting Calmness, and Comforting Encouraging?

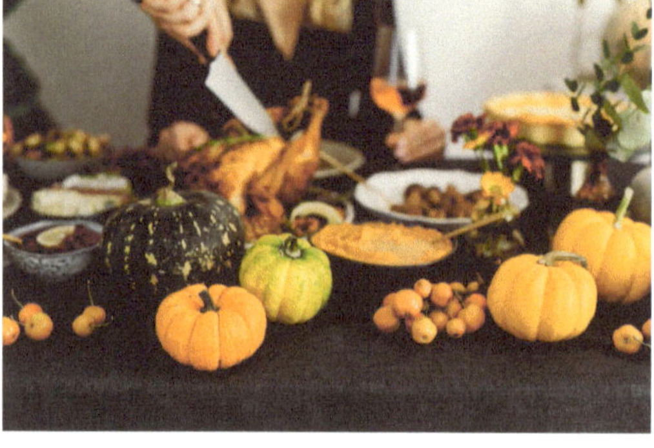

Indeed, whether the food is Turkey, Turkey Loaf, Chicken, or even rice and beans, the active ingredient in the Thanksgiving Dinner may well be the "TLC" component – the Tender Loving Care we experience – and the Turkey – aka the pharmaceutical – could be more of a placebo, or "filler"?

Might we ask, too: did Grandma learn how to be kind, supportive, soothing, from a School called the Turkey Dinner with TLC School, or from a book by the same name?

Indeed, for coffee drinkers or soda drinkers, the active or medicinal component might be the caffeine; and the flavors and the bubbles, and the chilled liquid, mere "fillers", placebo components, or what have you.

So, we ask, "Which components of healing are the medicine, and which are the fillers, the flavors, the fizz, the placebo components? Is it the chemicals, or the person administering the chemicals – the fillers?

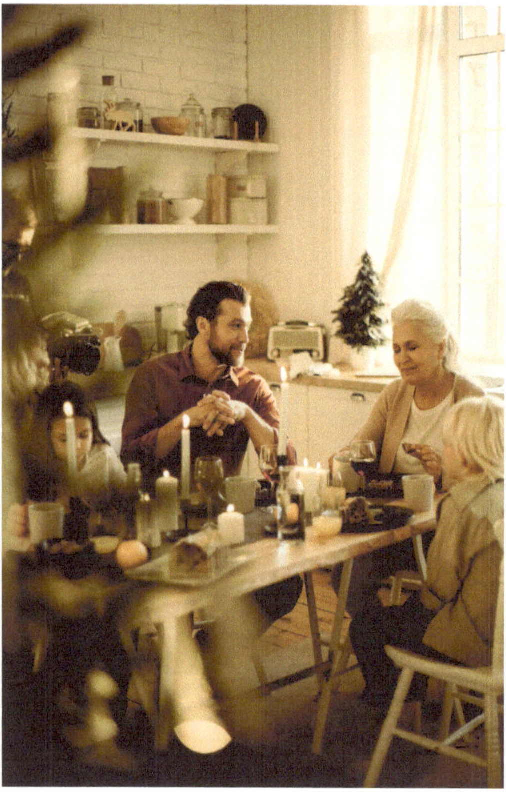

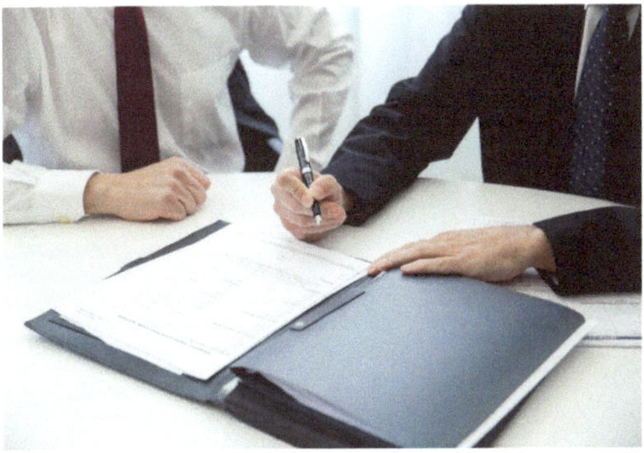

Grandma's accountant wants to know, was that one or two pieces of pumpkin pie, as part of the itemized bill you will receive, for services rendered.

This seems rather like the difference between having a good talk with a person, rather than watching someone have a good talk, on the television; one is more the medicine, the other, more like a filler: both have effects, but one is arguably far more potent than the other.

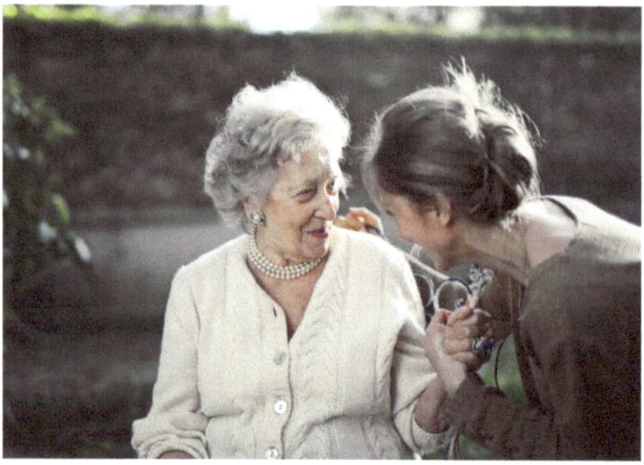

Want to be here, or see me on the Fac-simile Box?

We might even put it this way: which is the active ingredient; the emotions and words – perhaps referred to as the "Bedside Manner" Treatment; or, the other components administered alongside?

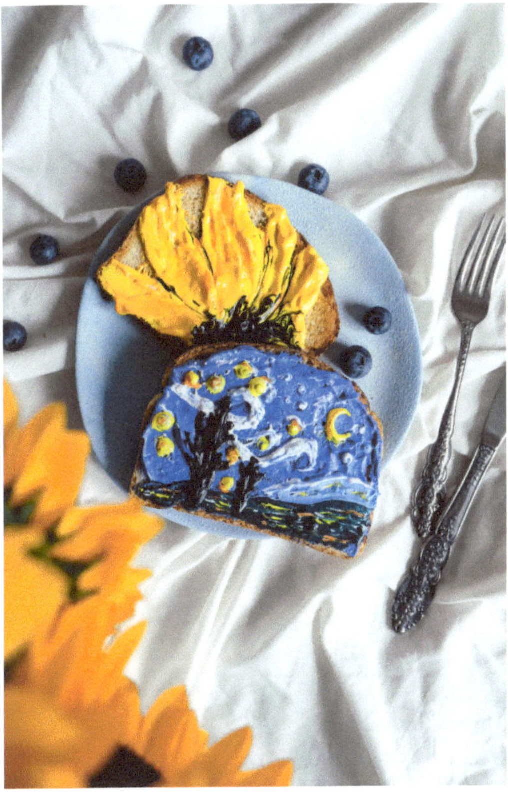

Is Grandma the active ingredient, or the apron she is wearing, and whether it was neatly pressed that day?

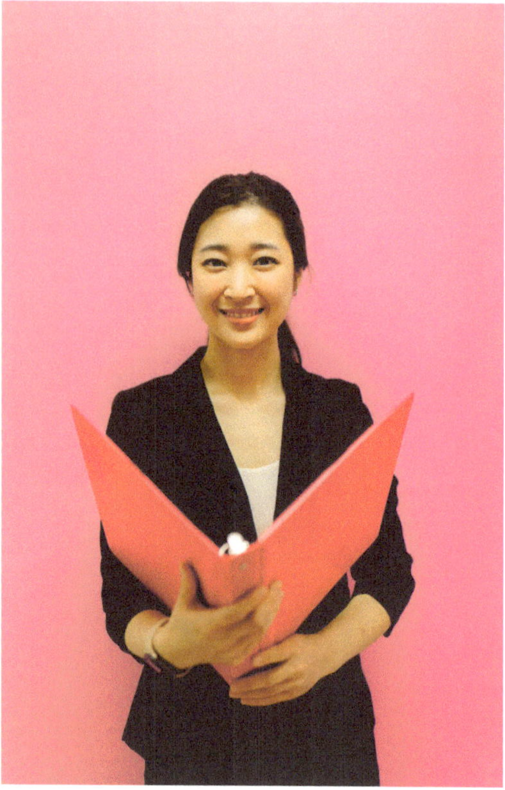

Did grandma forget to provide a spoon for your soup?

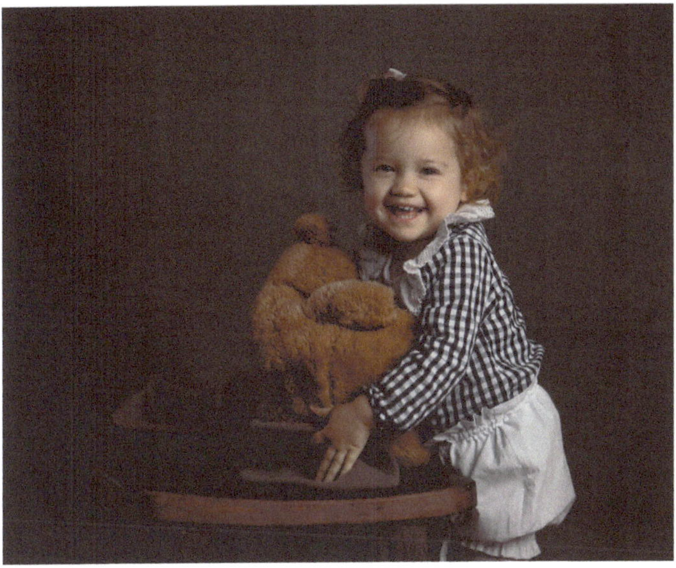

Chapter 7

We might ponder a few ideas from ship lore:

If a captain of a ship panics, during a storm, the crew members are also likely to panic, too, and the ship could then go down.

Or, too, if we could do the opposite – induce the opposite of panicking – induce soothing, instead – soothing of fears – might this be the active ingredient so direly needed?

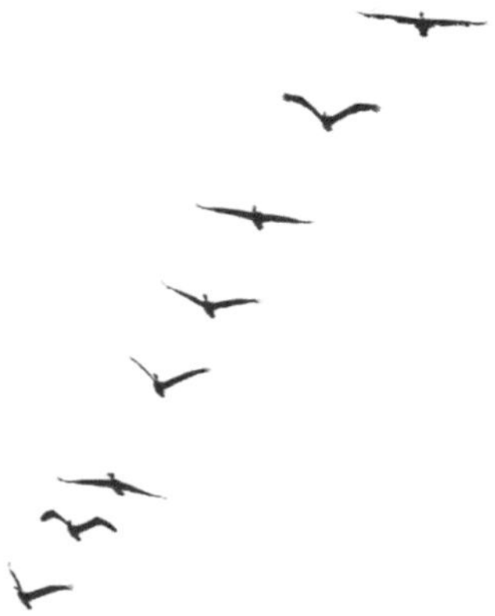

It'll come out in the wash, most likely!

Now, the ultimate in helping feel less anger and fear, is a lasting solution, not a temporary one.

We have heard the phrase, for instance, “I can give you a fish, or teach you to fish for yourself”

– the former is rather temporary, but the latter, more permanent.

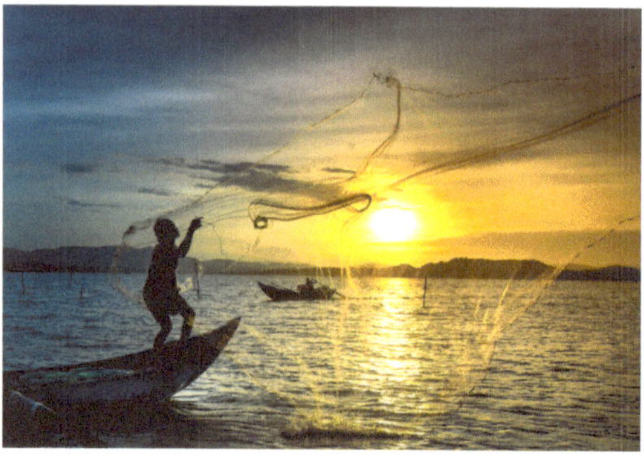

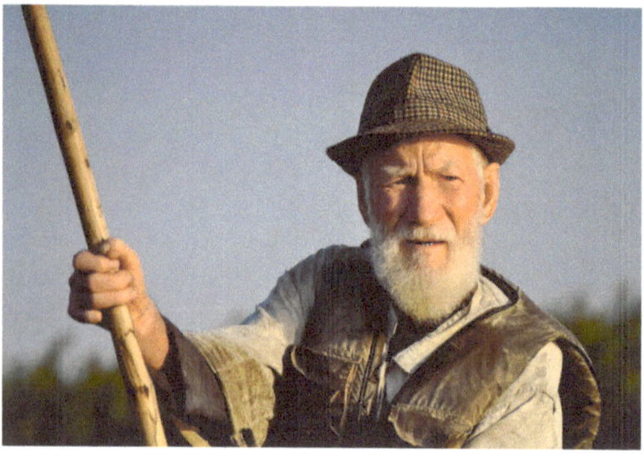

Likewise, if we are hard-working, and supportive of others, and seek to understand others as best we can, this could be, by far, very helpful in generating monetary income, whether or not the job market is going well or not.

Many a job place is so direly seeking such a person, that even if it ordinarily says they are "not hiring", they just might invent a new position title for the person who they would so desire to have on board.

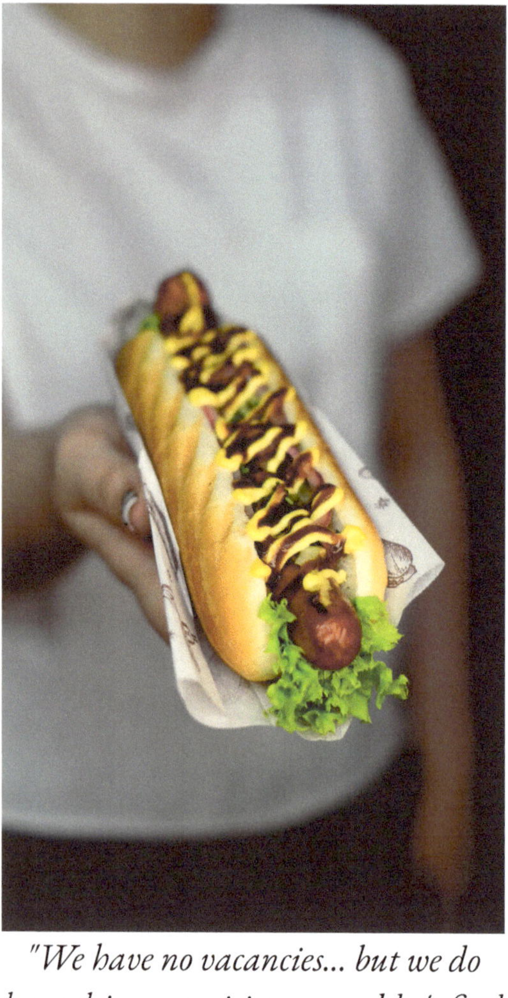

"We have no vacancies... but we do have this one position we couldn't find anyone to fill ... The Cheer-Meister: salary, $250,000. We were waiting for the right person to come along..."

We might refer to such, in the movies, as actors and actresses with "star quality".

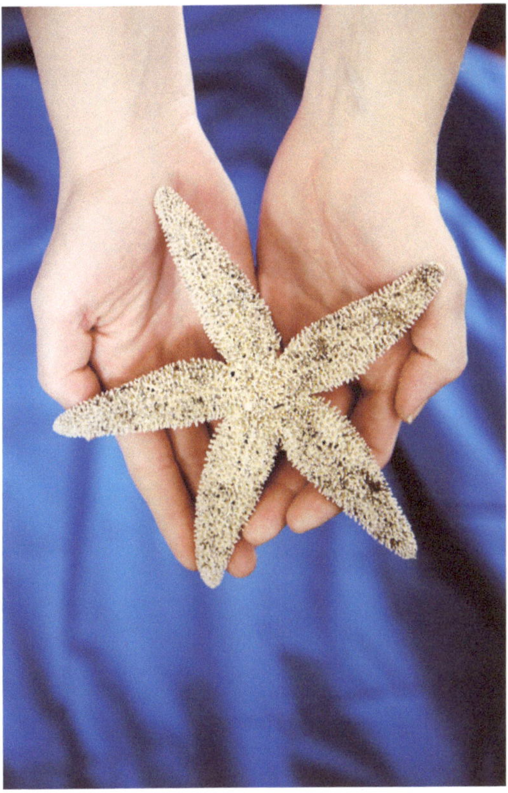

Furthermore, dating coaches are often urging people to pay great heed to their weight, grooming, and have their finances look appealing, also: with one exception.

For the person of Star Quality, the rules no longer apply; the Special Sauces, if you will, markedly transcend all else. Suddenly, the person of Star Quality can show up, wearing a tattered pair of jeans, a stained T-shirt, balding hair, a few or more extra pounds, be very non-muscular, short, and yet steal the entire show. Heads turn, and the phrase is, "Who is that person?" We cease to wonder about their financial portfolio, their age, their clothing, their cars, and their degrees and job titles. We simply say, "Wow".

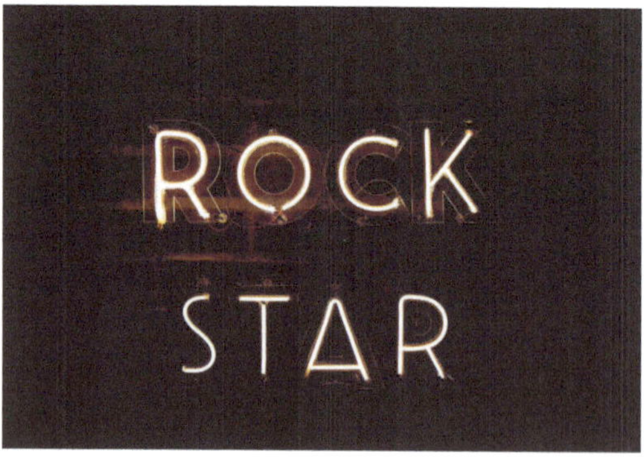

Mr. or Ms. WOW: no uniform required. Name your own hours.

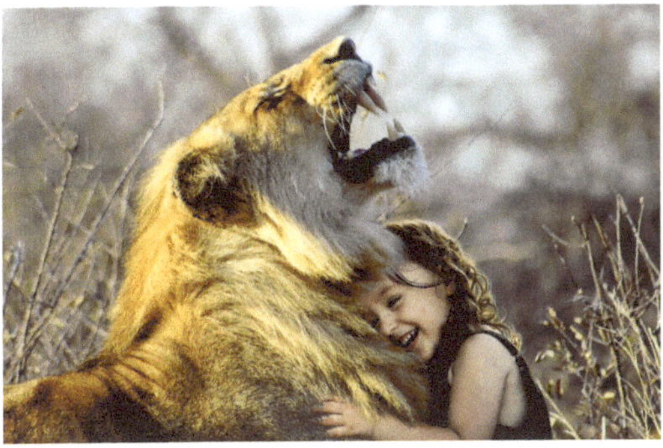

Who is that person? Who can turn adversity into silver linings?

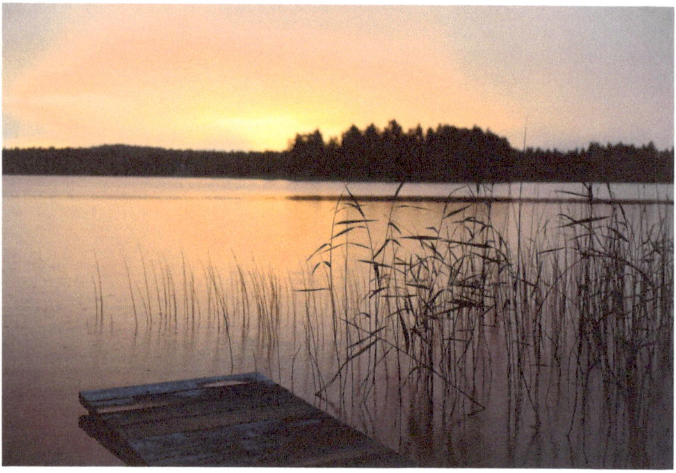

Chapter 8

The point being, perhaps all those former qualities are the Placebo Qualities, whereas the other, the Star Qualities, are the Medicine.

The Grandma Medicine. The TLC Medicine. The Catalyst Medicine. The Charisma Medicine. The Saint Medicine. The Inspiration Medicine. All else is Window Dressing or Perfume?

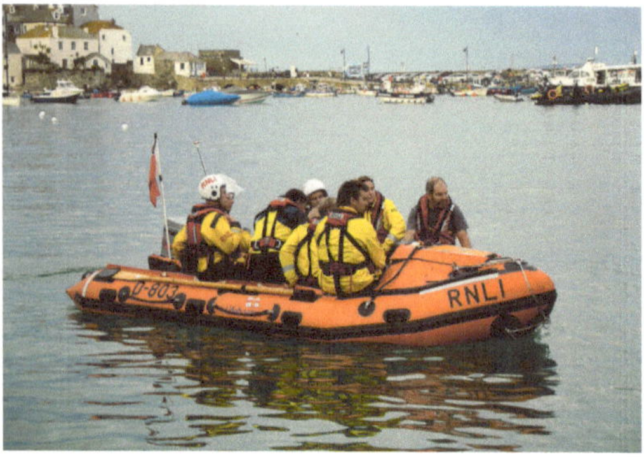

Will much of our medicinal approaches treat the problem, or try to rescue us?

We might analogize, too, that machines can keep us alive for long periods of time; so too, medicines of a chemical nature; but can either of these, change our words, our thoughts, our emotions, in turn?

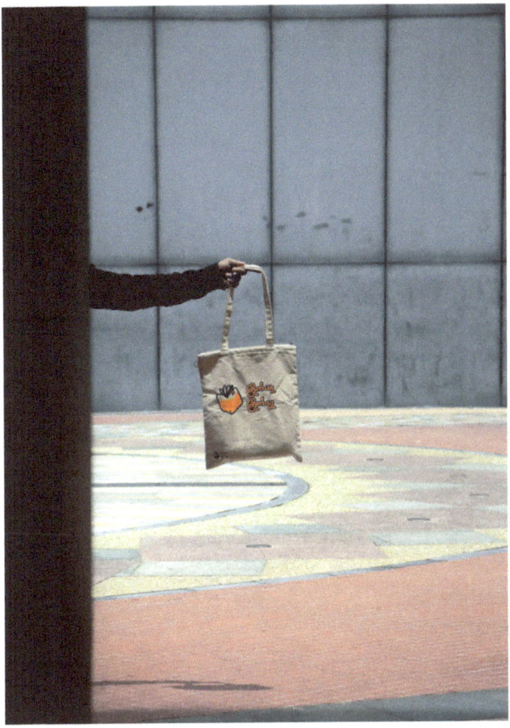

"Here's your medicine; now, I have to run, sorry; have a board meeting."

Does a frame make that much difference, or does the painting, when we are talking about a Picasso or Van Gogh? Are we also overly concerned over the lighting or the temperature of the air in the museum, as we view such?

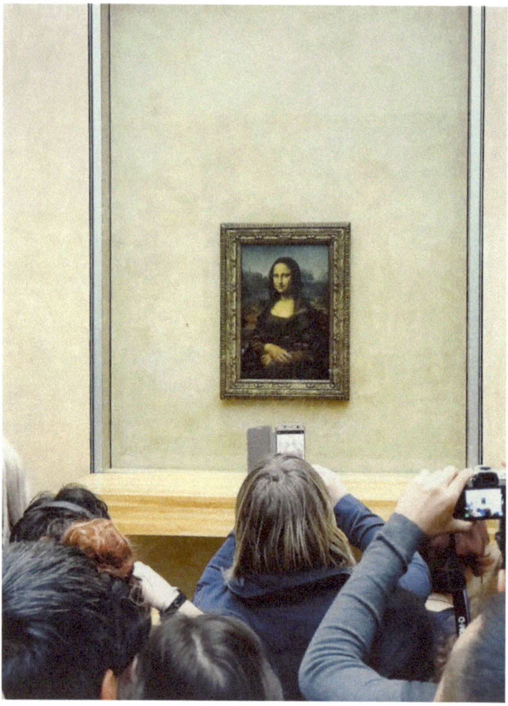

If we have a favorite ice cream, are we concerned with the color or shape of the carton it comes in? Or which store sold it? We want the active ingredient, the ice cream, and the inert ingredient, the placebo, if you will, is the filler, the "vehicle".

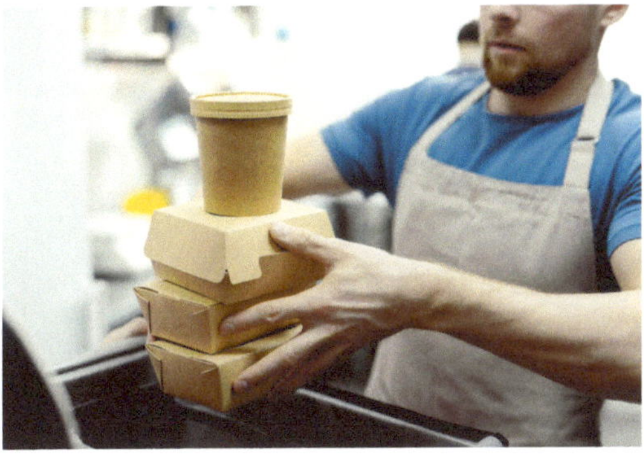

"Sorry, the colors on these boxes don't quite match, so we were almost going to cancel your order so that you wouldn't be upset..."

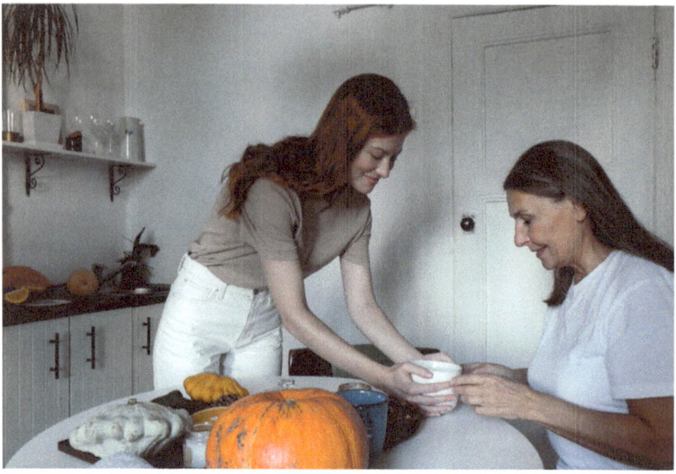

Chapter 9

So, we debate: are we to choose between Conventional Medicine, or Alternative Medicine? Or Religion? Or a vacation? Or a new job or spouse, or a new home or new living location, or perhaps have another child?

Are we to seek treatment by a medical doctor, or some other practitioner such as per Reiki, music therapy, art therapy, homeopathy, herbalism, and so on?

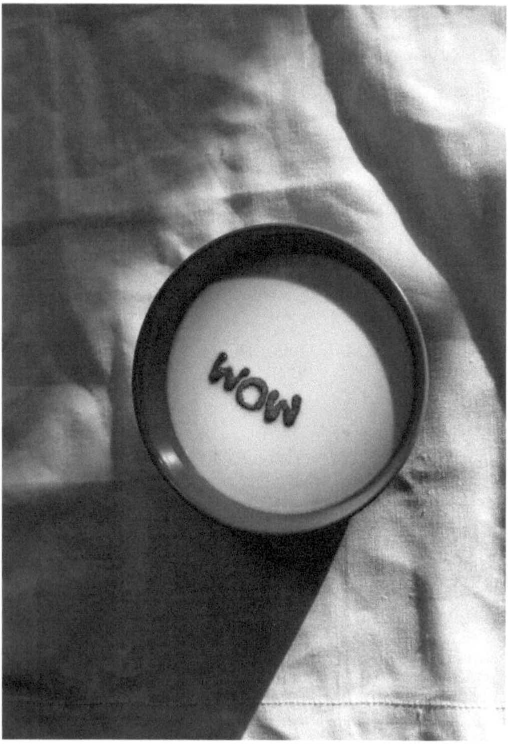

"How much for the WOW Medicine"?

Perhaps the choice is not clear-cut, one way or the other, because the number of persons in any of these areas who are able to administer the Truer Medicine, do not "Grow on Trees".

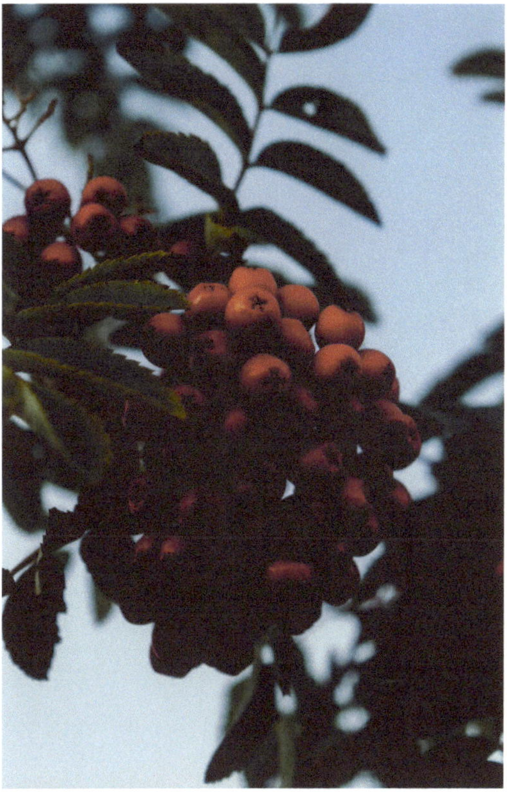

If medicine grows on trees, I must be looking in the wrong place?

Perhaps we need to invent a term for a third approach to treating our physical ailments, thus: a third option to Conventional or Alternative treatments:

Perhaps we need the treatment called "Star Quality" Medicine, in which our anger and fears are treated, via the modification of our thoughts, in turn.

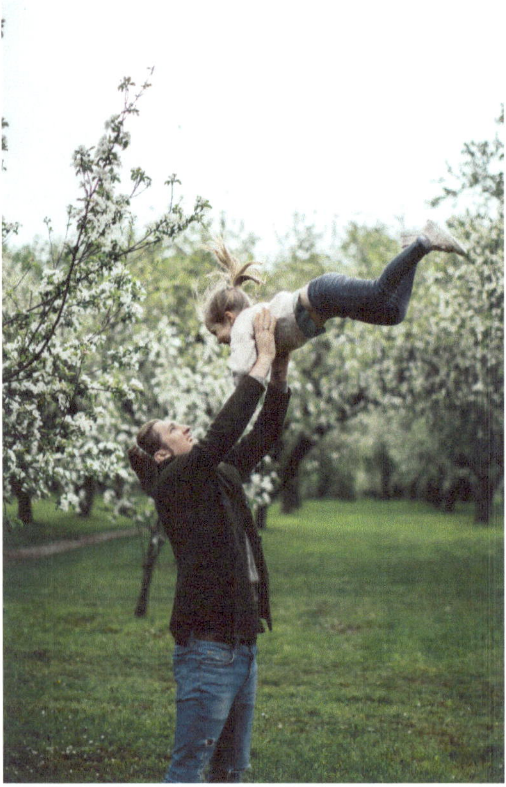

TLC Medicine, not THC or Meds-icine?

This does not appear to be regularly happening, some would say, in a therapy setting. If if were, we would see lines a mile or two long, at midnight, outside some therapy offices. In turn, we would all have heard of this.

There would, in turn, be a marked reduction in suffering. But this surely has not, in fact, happened. It would appear that we have word, or thought, therapy, in the rough, but not in the hand.

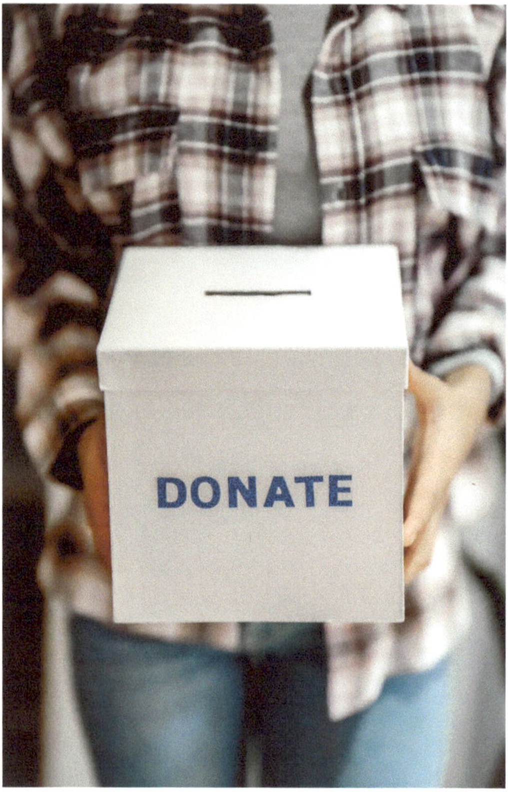

The box outside our therapist's door is for donations to defray the cost of their analyst?

***

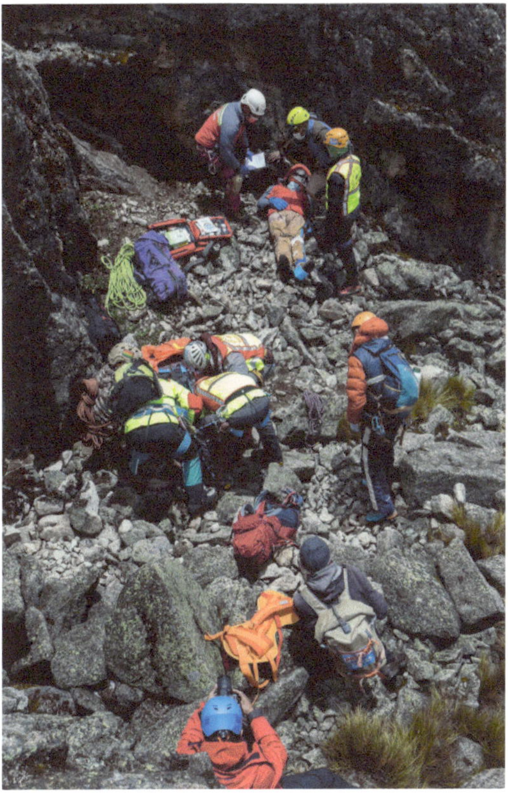

We repair what you tried to fix?

We have motions made, to alter our thinking for the better, but somehow, the outcome does not appear to match.

It thus appears, that personal growth takes time. The reduction of anger and fear, as part of personal growth, thus takes time.

Rome was not built in a day.

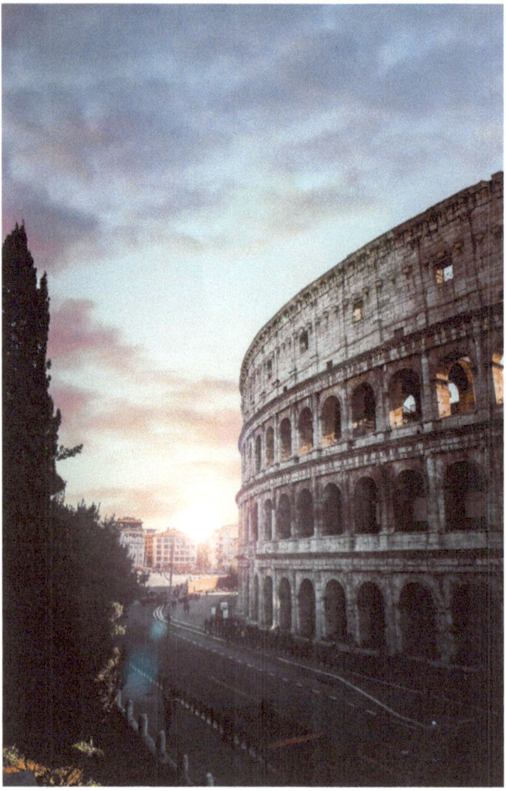

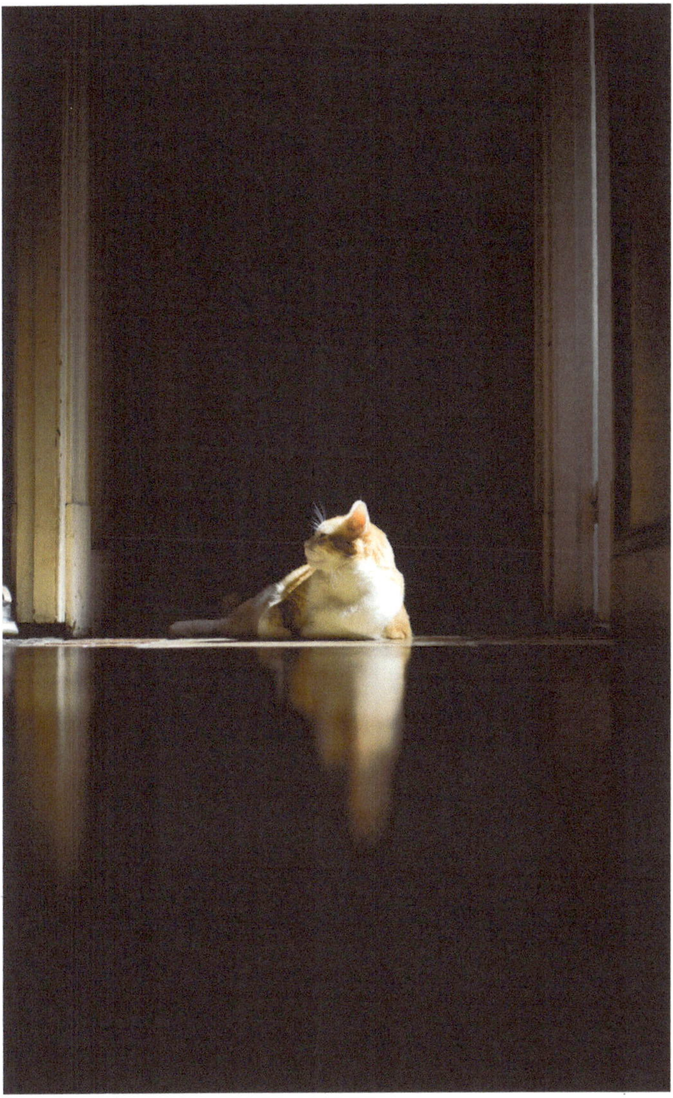

Chapter 10

So, to conclude, are we confusing the Modality with the Medicine, because the actual Medicine is not easy to come by?

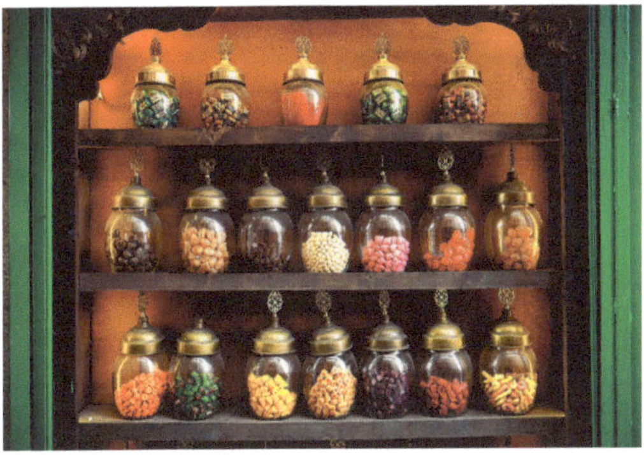

"Which color medicine did you want? Oh, you wanted a different container entirely? Sorry, that will have to be special-order..."

Does this medicine have to be created, ourselves? Is this what is meant by taking charge of our lives, and in turn, taking charge of our health? Does this entail, in turn, the taking charge of our anger and fear, in turn? Rather than hoping for some magic bullet pill or therapy treatment?

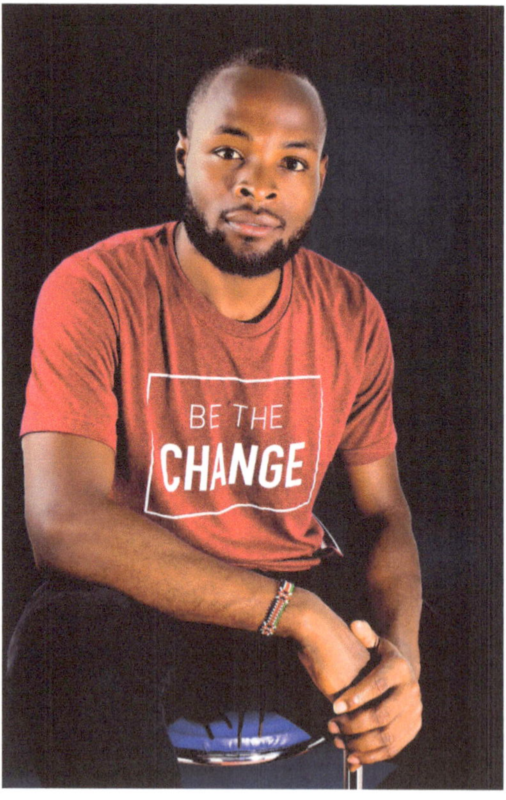

In closing, I make mention, the phrase by a childhood friend of mine: "If you want the job done right, you have to do it yourself".

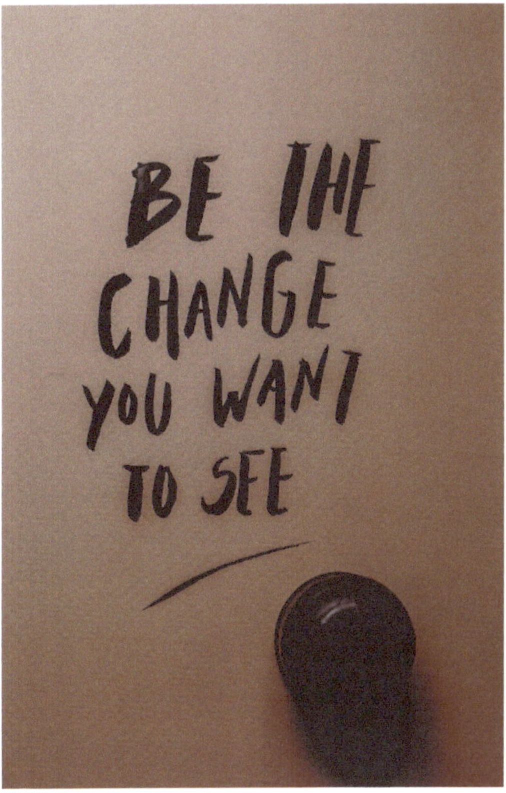

Might this also pertain to our own health, and our anger and fear, as key components?

As Jim Roan put it, to paraphrase: The Cavalry are not coming to rescue us.

It looks like we must rescue ourselves.

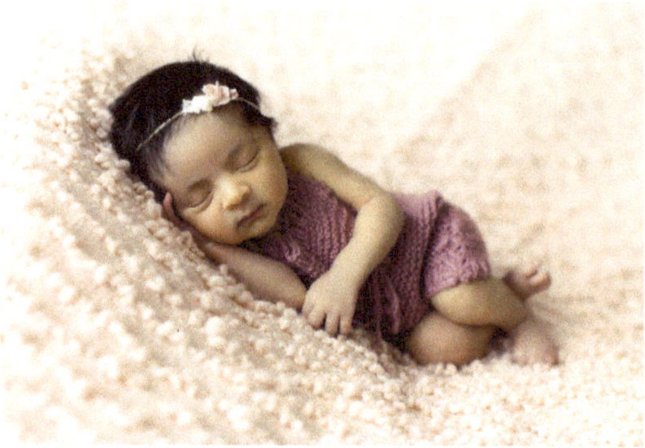

The cavalry are still asleep?

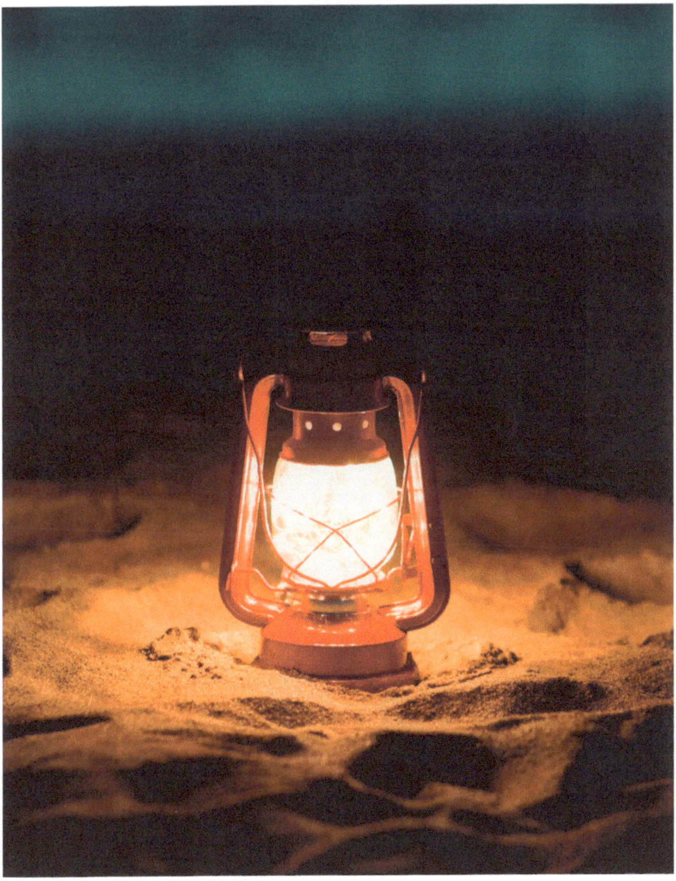

Chapter II: Example of a Healing Archetype? A Movie on YouTube

The following movie, exemplifies a type of healer, perhaps:

The Last Passport: Award-Winning Feature Film

https://youtu.be/h-axJKVYbmk

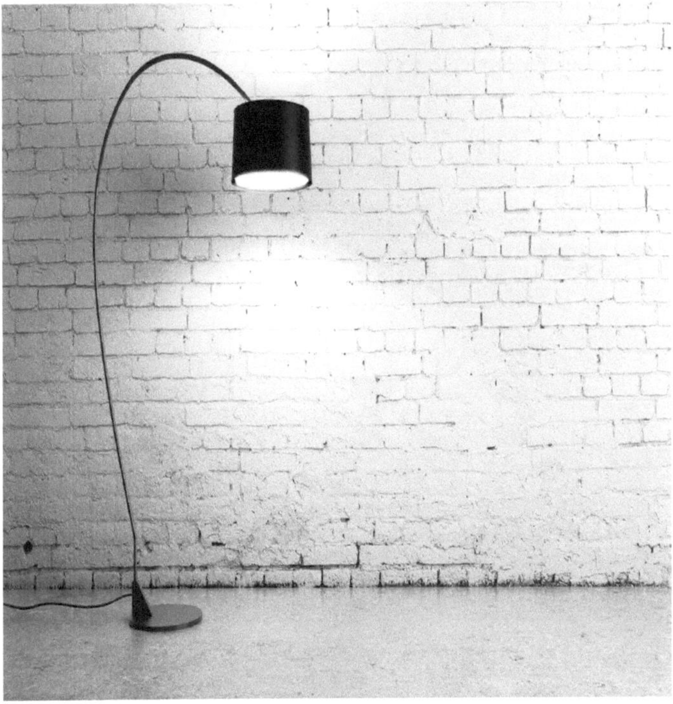

Finale: Not Everything is Rocket Science

Perhaps not everything is rocket science?

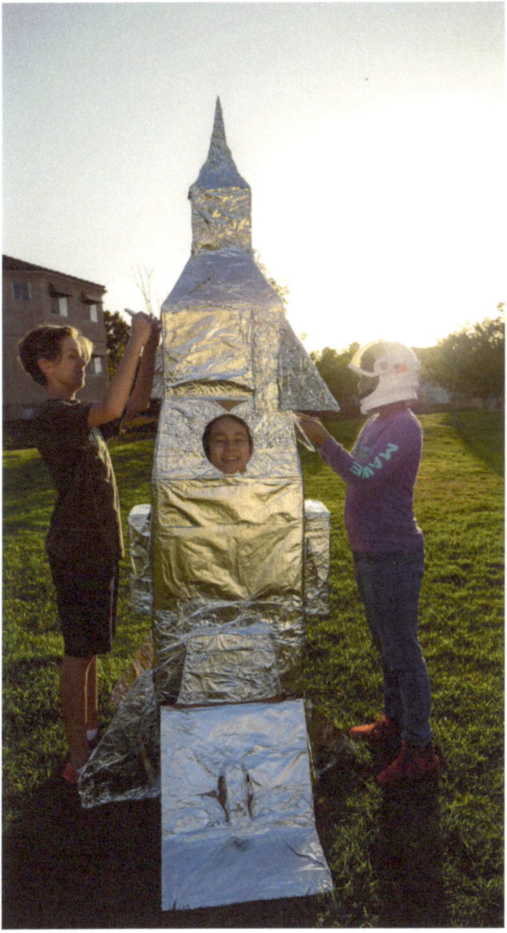

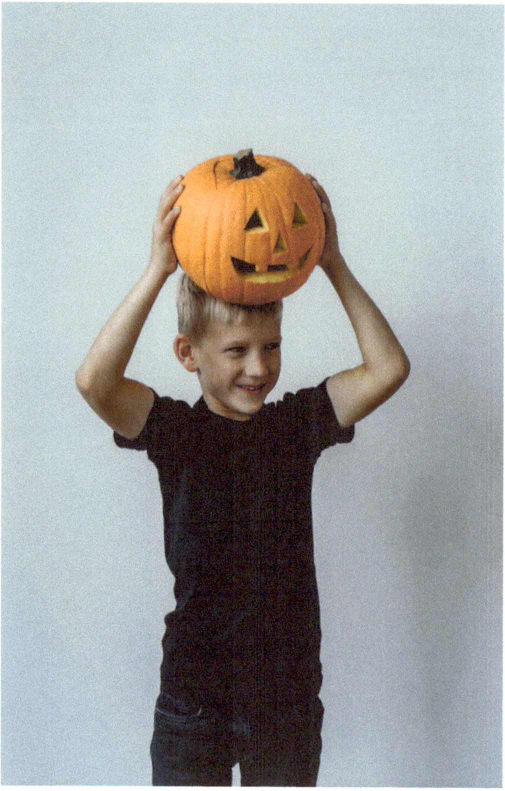

Time to grab the pumpkin by the horns?

A final word:

The following quotation has been attributed to the writer and political commentator Gore Vidal:

"The four most beautiful words in the English language are 'I told you so'."

https://quoteinvestigator.com/2015/12/11/told/

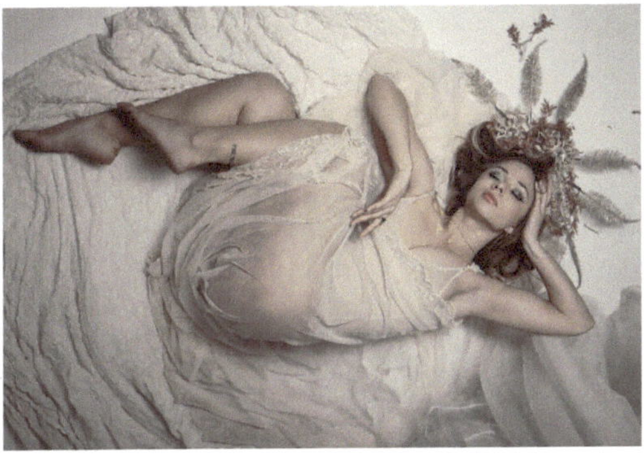

But surely you're joking, right?

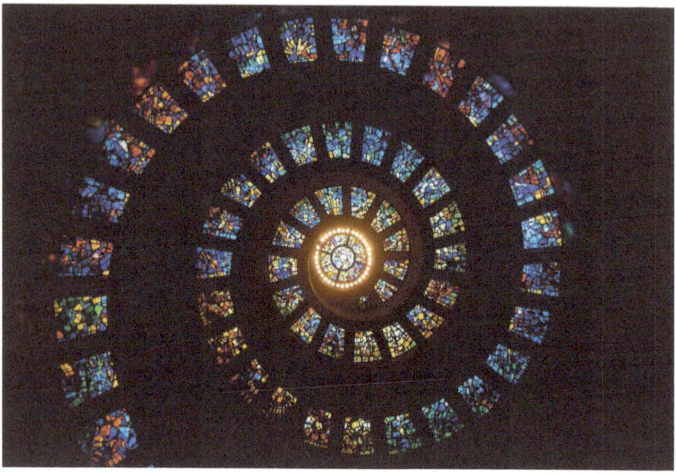

To the thinkers
of the world,
including Jacques Cousteau,
one of the few television programs
my parents vetted for my viewing,
when I was a youth:
"The Fascinating Underwater World
and the Legacy of Jacques Cousteau":
https://youtu.be/KKC3MTgzZeM

**"Jacques Cousteau was a French undersea explorer, researcher, photographer and documentary host
who invented diving and scuba devices, including the Aqua-Lung."**

https://www.biography.com/history-culture/jacques-cousteau

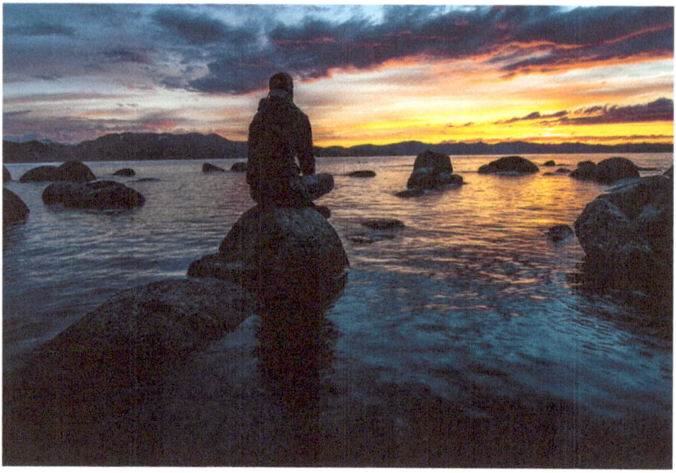

HEALTH CARE TODAY: EXPANDED EDITION

Video and Print Resources

A few curiosities...

1.Who is to say exactly what is or isn't the active ingredient to a useful approach?

Might we consider:

1. "The Magic of Marie Laveau: Embracing the Spiritual Legacy of the Voodoo Queen of New Orleans".

"**Marie Laveau** ... born 1801?, New Orleans, Louisiana – died June 15, 1881, New Orleans) was the Vodou queen of New Orleans. Laveau's powers reportedly included healing the sick, extending altruistic gifts to the poor, and overseeing spiritual rites."

https://www.britannica.com/biography/Marie-Laveau

2. "The best teacher I ever had", by Bill Gates

https://youtu.be/WOoJh6oYAXE

"Feynman was basically the Bruce Lee of physics."

@ThaReaChuckD

3. "Feynman: Take the world from another point of view (1/4)"

https://youtu.be/PsgBtOVzHKI

4. "Feynman : Knowing versus Understanding"

https://youtu.be/NM-zWTU7X-k

5. "Richard Feynman. Why."

https://youtu.be/36GT2zI8lVA

6. "(Brief) History of Norman Cousins"

https://youtu.be/t50r903AeHY

7. "'Sick Boy' Lives In Sterilized Bubble For 18 Years"

A man born without an immune system starts living life inside a physical bubble. When he learns that the girl whom he loves is about to get married, he builds a portable bubble to get to her.□

https://youtu.be/qQPyEsgQVio

8. "When You Think For Yourself or Follow The Crowd"

https://youtu.be/lEp45b3n4F0

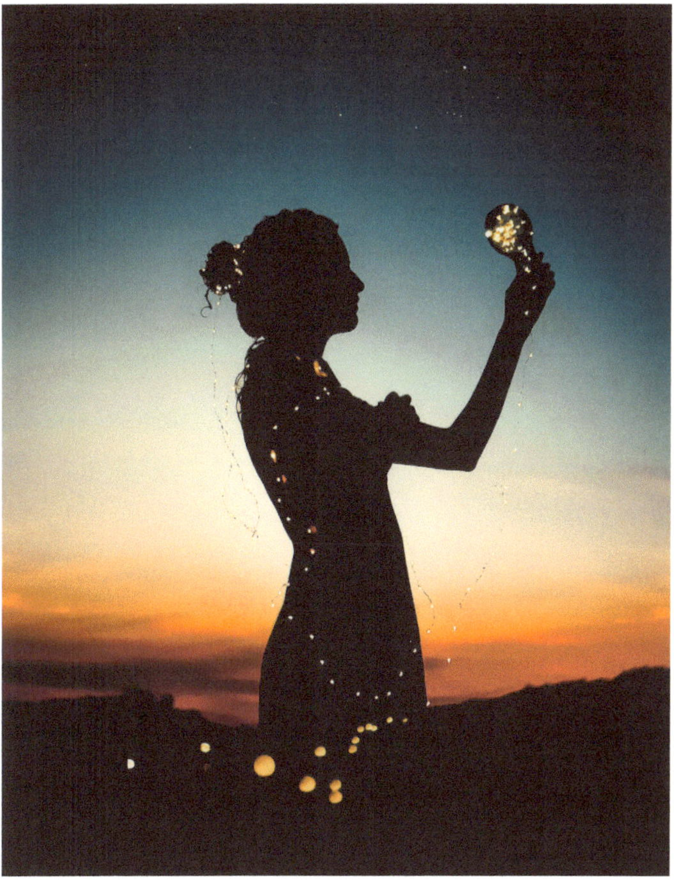

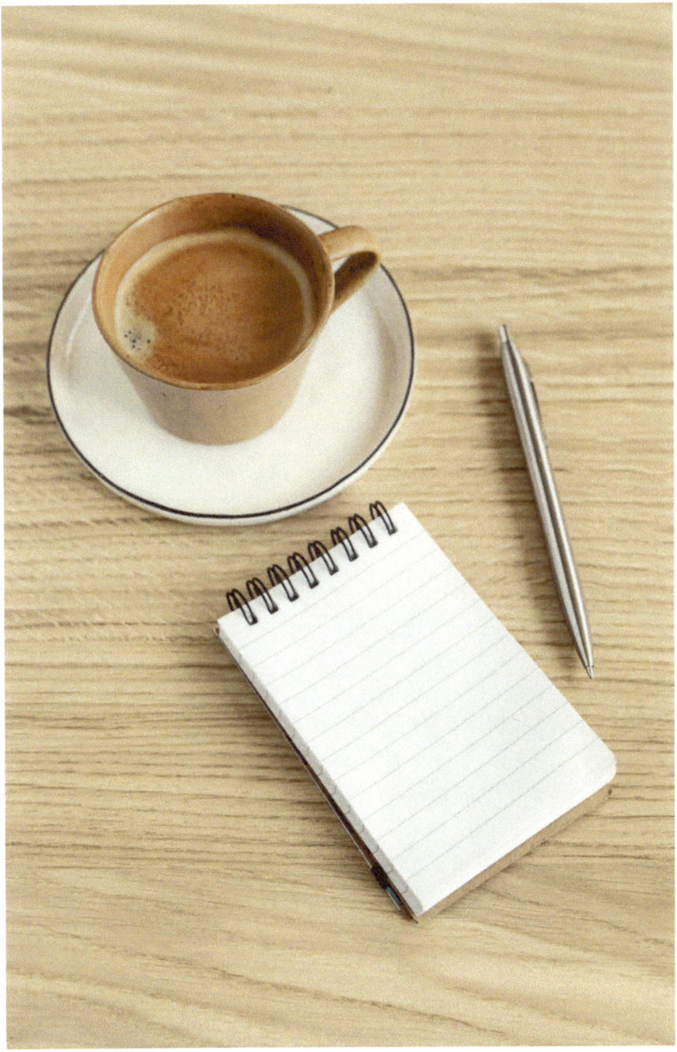

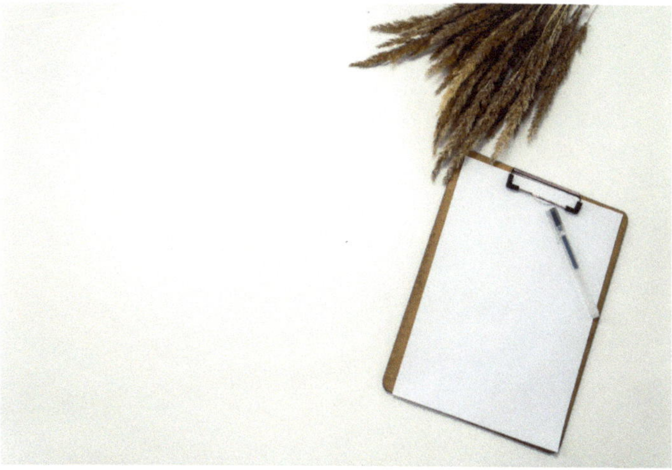

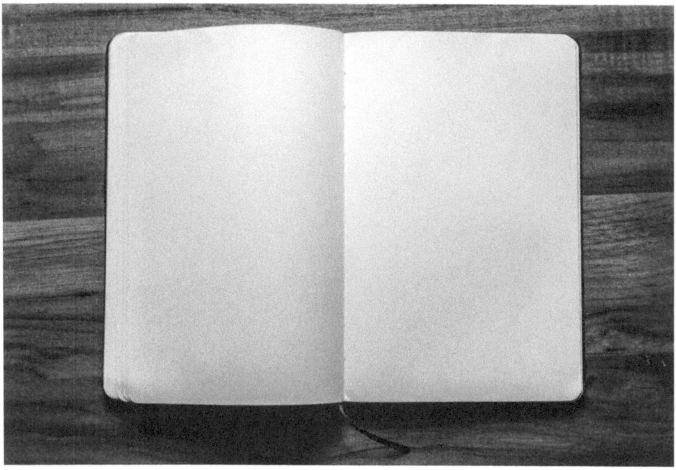

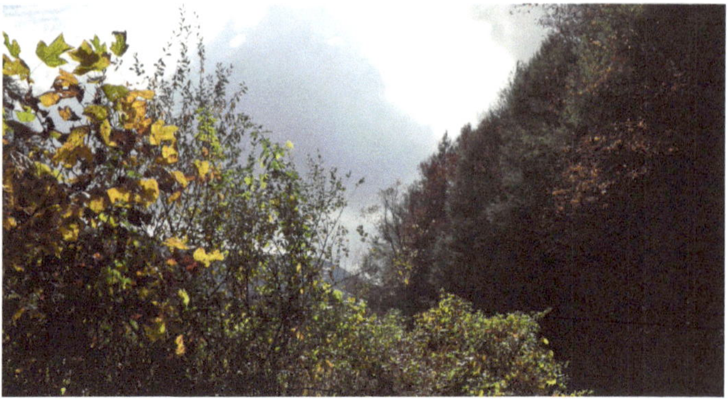

www.ingramcontent.com/pod-product-compliance
Ingram Content Group UK Ltd.
Pitfield, Milton Keynes, MK11 3LW, UK
UKHW061538051026
15625UKWH00009B/510
* 9 7 9 8 3 4 8 3 6 7 2 8 2 *